Micro Miracle

Micro Miracle

A True Story

Amy Boyes

Signature
EDITIONS

Cover design by Doowah Design.
Photo of Amy Boyes by Eva Wong.

This book was printed on Ancient Forest Friendly paper.
Printed and bound in Canada by Marquis Book Printing Inc.

We acknowledge the support of the Canada Council for the Arts and the Manitoba Arts Council for our publishing program.

Library and Archives Canada Cataloguing in Publication

Boyes, Amy, 1985-, author
        Micro miracle : a true story / Amy Boyes.

Issued in print and electronic formats.
ISBN 978-1-77324-037-4 (softcover).--ISBN 978-1-77324-038-1 (EPUB)

        1. Boyes, Amy, 1985-. 2. Mothers of prematurely born children--Canada--Biography. 3. Premature infants--Canada--Biography.
4. Premature infants--Care. I. Title.

RJ250.B694 2018   618.92'011092   C2018-905148-5
                                                 C2018-905149-3

Signature Editions
P.O. Box 206, RPO Corydon, Winnipeg, Manitoba, R3M 3S7
www.signature-editions.com

To Madeline
I hope you feel my love on every page

Introduction

MOST BABIES BORN SIXTEEN WEEKS EARLY ARE NOT EXPECTED TO survive without disabilities or developmental delays. Although outcomes for extremely premature infants have improved dramatically in recent years, even today, 40–50% of infants born fourteen to fifteen weeks early will die shortly after birth. Of the remainder, as many as 75% will suffer disabilities and delays (Morse, Zheng, Tang, & Roth, 2009; Petrini et al., 2009).

In many countries, maternal and infant health care suffers from inadequate funding and resources. Costs for months of hospitalization, testing, and surgeries can quickly reach into the hundreds of thousands. Even in some developed countries, parents have to consider their insurance and health care benefits when deciding whether to resuscitate a premature infant or allow the infant to pass away without intervention. In Canada, public health care eliminates the need for private insurance or work-place health benefits for primary care.

This story is an example of how the smallest, most fragile citizen is valued in a civilized society. The essence of our humanity is shown by how we treat those who cannot help themselves, especially when the costs and risks are high.

SHE DOESN'T LOOK LIKE A BABY. SHE LOOKS LIKE A MISSING LINK between an embryo sketch and a wide-eyed Gerber baby. She has a complete assemblage of infant anatomy, yet she falters, functioning only at the pleasure of machines.

I read the birth record taped to her incubator as if it were a description on a museum display case:

Madeline Boyes
24 weeks gestational age
16 weeks premature
1 pound, 6 ounces, 12 inches long

I watch for signs of life, but there aren't any. Instead, I take the word of machines, beeping out evidence in long electronic lines, that she's alive.

She lies still, her wrinkled limbs flopped across a stiff flannel sheet. A sunshine-yellow toque covers her tennis ball–sized head. Her tiny bits of ears peek out from under the toque's fuzzy yarn. Cartilage hasn't formed yet, so her ears are just flaps of skin, folded forward against her head. Her puffy eyelids are fused together like a newborn kitten's. Their inability to open creates an illusion of blindness, a suggestion she'll never see the worried faces hovering over her. Saliva foams and dries around the ventilator tube that slinks over her pointed chin, into her gaping mouth. She has no fat, nothing to plump the pouches of skin that drip off her jaw and pile into layers on her neck and shoulders, just a coat of downy hair to protect against the amniotic fluid she no longer swims in. With each breath forced into her underdeveloped lungs by the mechanical ventilator, her ribs protrude against her crimson, gelatinous skin like shark fins skimming the surface of the ocean. Her fragility disturbs me. I'm overwhelmed by her helplessness.

I inhale deeply, trying to stop the room from spinning. Gripping the side of the incubator, I whisper through the Plexiglas pane that separates us, "I love you, Madeline."

She opens her mouth in a silent scream and claws at the air with thin fingers. She seems resentful of being ripped from the nurturing womb and plopped onto a drafty resuscitation table. She can't be cared for like other babies and she can't be put back where she came from. She's been pushed into the world and declared a baby, but I cannot accept the declaration. She's too wrinkled and half-formed. How will she survive? It isn't possible.

But in this dark, hushed ward, this endless cavern of incubators lit by a dozen machines all churning out life, a steely-nerved nurse takes my shaking hands, stares into my exhausted eyes, and says calmly, "Good evening, Mrs. Boyes, and welcome to the Neonatology Intensive Care Unit. I understand you've just given birth. I know she's a bit of shock, but she's your baby. She's your Madeline."

Chapter 1

ONE AUGUST AFTERNOON, THE SUMMER BEFORE, I SET OFF ON the Katimavik footpath. Although the Ottawa Greenbelt has other paths, paths that can compete for solitude and scenery with those of the Gatineau Hills or the Adirondack Mountains, we residents of suburban Kanata are content to walk the cracked pavement which lies behind our own backyards. Maybe busy residents appreciate the path for its closeness, freeing them from driving to remote parking lots; sociable residents, for the ease with which new acquaintances can be made, a quick hello turning into a lifelong friendship; and dog-walking residents, for the aromatic garbage bins which overflow with bulging plastic bags tied in elaborate knots.

I like to walk the path in a wide, four-kilometre loop. Perhaps other regulars recognize me by my blonde ponytail swinging from side to side or by my gaudy fuchsia flip-flops slapping the asphalt. Indeed, recognizing a fellow path-walker is almost as affirming as having your Toronto cousin breeze into town and compliment you on your toned calves. You're assured of your own discipline much more pleasantly than if you simply checked off a box on an unwieldy exercise chart.

When I begin my walk, the sun is already sinking. There's no reason why I didn't go earlier—I'm on summer holiday from teaching and had spent the day as I pleased—but the day had been warm, so I delayed my walk until leaves rustled with a hint of breeze and long shadows formed.

Summer in Ottawa can be oppressive. Unlike the dry prairie heat I grew up with, Ottawa's heat sits heavily, damp and suffocating. But the ferocity of summer is mirrored by the unpleasantness of winter, and the knowledge that summer will soon end drives me out of our air-conditioned house and onto the footpath.

The footpath has no obvious design. It's just a series of inter-connected trails that were paved during a decade of residential development. It begins close to our house, under a power line, and weaves around faded play structures, boulders landscaped into the general impression of Stonehenge, and weathered wooden benches built low to the ground, initialled by *les enfants terribles* long since fled from the suburbs. Every so often, the path pops out of park-land to cross a street. But mostly the path is sheltered from staring, bored residents bobbing on backyard pool floats by a corridor of dogwoods, elms, and maples. Between the trees, light-deprived wild-flowers spring up on gangly stems while, here and there, crisp leaves anticipate autumn, wafting down to the path below. It's a peaceful path, a respite from the city within the city.

I occasionally dare myself to jog, albeit never for very long. I want to be reasonably fit, but without too much exertion. How I am to balance slothfulness and fitness, I haven't considered, but daily walks seem like a good idea. As a consistent size six, I naively believe I can take a cavalier approach to fitness, leaving the hard work for those that wander the racks of Addition Elle.

If asked why I walk, I might refer to the benefits of fresh air and sunshine. But as I flip-flop down the path, the late afternoon sun speckling gold shadows over the charcoal pavement, I consider my other reason for walking: I want a baby—a bright-eyed, rosy-cheeked baby—and I want a strong body to carry it in. I've read magazine articles about labour and the "post-pregnancy body," and they all encourage a pre-pregnancy fitness regime. The baby is healthier and the mother is happier. Labour might even be easier. So I walk and, as I walk, I think about a baby.

I've always imagined I'd be a mother at some point in my life. Childbearing seems inevitable, like finishing a degree or planning for retirement. It's what people do and, viewed from a distance, the process seems reasonable.

My husband Josh and I spent the first years of our marriage ignor-ing our parents' sly inquiries after grandchildren, confining our own discussions of babies to quiet whispers while drifting off to sleep or quick quips while speed-walking past the playground. Although we liked the idea of a baby, a cheerful cherub straight from the Pampers ads—who wouldn't?—we had a mortgage and careers to consider. But now, we're two and half years into our marriage. He works as an assistant to a Member of Parliament in the House of Commons; I, as a music teacher. We've saved some money. We have a house with a wee yard. We're over the worst of the nitpicky scrappiness that accompanies any two people sharing a roof for the first time, and we're both near thirty. It's as good a time as any to have a baby—why not?

But as I rest on a bench for a minute and watch the leaves drift and float, I'm struck by how presumptuous the idea feels. By deciding to create a life, we're also assuming we have the talents and skills necessary to nurture a life. From that perspective, having a child seems audacious, arrogant even. Why do we imagine we're qualified to raise a child?

My parents had kids though. And their parents too. They don't seem to regret it. In fact, they seem sure of themselves, confident, authoritative. They always have the answers to life's questions. They're not riddled with self-doubt. Besides, if they and everyone else thought as hard about having children as I'm thinking, the earth's population would cease to grow. Every responsible, sane person would look over the brink and back away carefully. No one would commit themselves to such risk-taking. For what else is childbearing but supreme risk-taking?

My mom, a no-nonsense farm wife, would say having children was the natural thing to do. "Just get on with it"—I can hear her voice in my head—"People have kids. It's what we do." And she's probably right. The wisdom of her advice is evidenced by its simplicity.

I listen to the sounds of a neighbourhood returning from work, cooking suppers, walking dogs. The sounds are innocuous and fragmented but, put together, the car doors slamming, the cannonballs splashing, and the barbeque lids thumping are all part of life, one day after another. There's a comfort in these sounds, in the momentum that carries us from one year to the next, from one generation to another. Our lives wouldn't be the same without little people running through them. Audacious or not, Josh and I would always regret not having a child. Despite my qualms, I know it.

I pick a crunchy oak leaf off my shoulder and walk on, toward the curve in the trail that will eventually lead me home.

• • •

IT DOESN'T TAKE LONG FOR THE HEAT OF AUGUST TO DISAPPEAR. Winter comes, swift and sure as it always does, and as the days grow shorter I have suspicions. One morning in early November, I tear the packaging off a test strip and proceed as directed on the side of the pink box: "Insert into cup for five seconds. Wait three minutes."

It doesn't take three minutes. One pink line instantly appears and, a moment later, another line faintly traces across the screen. Half the width of the first, the second line is the life-changer. Apparently, I'm pregnant.

I stare at my reflection in the toothpaste-spotted mirror, half expecting a Madonna-like halo to form above my head. I feel peace and panic, both at once. The long-awaited game is on, and I already feel a shift in my thinking. It's as if I've stepped out of one section of a timeline into another, like Mozart in the textbooks, launching the Classical era, leaving the Baroque behind. I am leaving the land of carefree maidens, venturing somewhere new, somewhere with curvaceous women and general exhaustion.

When Josh comes home from work, I meet him at the door and with the tiniest bit of nervousness whisper my news.

"Oh, Babe," he sighs and grins like he knew all along. He pulls me close and I lay my head on his shoulder. "You're going to make a wonderful mother," he whispers, kissing my neck, wiping his eyes.

"It's hard to imagine!" I laugh and then call myself, for the very first time, "Mom."

Chapter 2

THERE'S BLOOD.

Eight weeks pregnant and there's blood. There isn't much, but it doesn't take much blood to cause alarm. A little smudge, a little pink. Mostly pale. Watered down. Maybe it's innocent, but I feel panic.

I've had a rough start to my pregnancy. Every morning, noon, and occasionally night, I throw up into a water pitcher, gripping the handle as the contents of my stomach splash below. Then I lie still, breathing softly, savouring ten minutes of stillness before the wretchedness begins again.

One day, early in my pregnancy, I decided there had to be a cure for the misery and went online to find it. But throughout the last hundred years, so many typewriters and keyboards have punched out words of advice to the pregnant that the resulting wisdom is a tangled web of nonsense. Indeed, the astronomical number of results that popped onto my screen when I searched Amazon for pregnancy guides made me want to swipe the laptop shut and take a nap. But I persevered, ordering a classic guide that has remained unchallenged on forty years of bestseller lists.

And when it arrived, two business days later, I flipped to the nausea section with anticipation, only to read that a few crackers and fresh air would soon set me right.

Unfortunately, I threw up before, during, and after those crackers. In fact, crackers seemed to only increase the ferocity of my vomiting. I gave up on crackers, tossed the pregnancy guide under the bed, and called my mother. She recommended chopped fruit, which I tried and promptly threw up. She then suggested a small glass of milk, which descended and ascended even before it lost its chill in my stomach.

I inquired of older friends, but discovered that women are mostly divided into two equally unhelpful camps. There are the deathly ill while pregnant who console you with—"Nothing works, dear. I threw up three times a day for nine months with all my four children. You hold on and wait for it to be over"—and the perky ones who had sunshine pregnancies—"I LOVED being pregnant! My skin was so soft and I had so much positive energy."

I decided it was hopeless and I just had to wait for time to pass, nauseated or not. But now time has passed.

It's December and there's blood. I consult the pregnancy guides and to my dismay find advice that runs the gamut from "Early bleeding is fairly common and is nothing to worry about," to "Half the women who bleed during the first twelve weeks eventually miscarry though not necessarily at the same time they experience bleeding." The more I read, the more variations on the theme of miscarriage emerge. It seems that every condition, every symptom has the potential to be lethal. But as the authors reach that mortal climax, the column comes to an end, the sidebar drops away, and the subject changes. Next chapter!

I watch the splotches for a day or two, worrying over them, wishing them away. Josh tries to comfort me: "It's likely nothing, Babe. These things happen." But since he doesn't know, and neither do I, I call my doctor, trying to sound like I have it all together.

"Is this anything to be concerned about?" I ask, my voice quavering.

"Don't stress!" my doctor replies cheerfully as "It's the Most Wonderful Time of the Year" plays in the background. "I'll send you for an ultrasound and if the cervix is strong and the heart is beating, you've got nothing to worry about!"

She doesn't sound alarmed; in fact, she sounds downright chirpy. But is it because my symptoms are no cause for concern or because she's getting ready to leave on her Christmas vacation? Still, as I hang up the phone, I feel like I have a better perspective on the situation. There are bigger worries than nausea; there is a fragile life to consider. Suddenly nothing feels guaranteed.

• • •

"FLOOR 4, ROOM 120," JOSH READS FROM THE APPOINTMENT CARD as we step inside a musty elevator. I press the "4" button until it partially lights up, obscured by half a century's worth of mildew.

The elevator is decorated for the season—artificial poinsettias, presumably flaming red at one time, now faded to dull terracotta; glossy tinsel garlands drooping from the ceiling; and a notice for the "Elvis Sighting Society Annual Christmas Day Dinner" posted on a corkboard. As the elevator thumps to a stop on the fourth floor, asthma and allergy patients track mud to an office on the left; we, to the Women's Ultrasound Clinic on the right.

The clinic's waiting room is filled with pregnant women wedged into narrow chairs. They calmly flip through the pages of *Chatelaine* and *Today's Parent* as their stomachs protrude beyond unbuttoned sweaters, straining even the forgiving elasticity of knit tops. I catch myself gaping, dreading the inevitable expansion of my own waist line.

Josh hangs our jackets on a portable coat rack. It's minus-twenty Celsius outside, bitter with a breeze, so the spindly rack is stuffed with heavy jackets. I lean on Josh's arm for balance as I unzip my winter boots then set them on a rubber tray encrusted with street salt, beside other similarly sensible footwear. My big toe emerges out a hole in of my tights, so I pick at the Lycra, trying to shift the hole to the bottom of my foot.

"How are you feeling?" Josh asks.

"Like it may not be anatomically possible to finish all this." I wave a one-litre water bottle.

"Three more guzzles and you'll have it down."

"I wonder where the washroom is," I say, peering around the waiting room.

A woman in her forties looks up from the magazine resting on her stomach. "Right beside the ultrasound room, dear. They know what they are doing." She smiles sympathetically. Perhaps she remembers her first ultrasound as a twenty-something and wishes it back.

We sit down and, after what feels like an eternity to my bladder, a technician with sad eyes and a Russian accent calls, "Ah-MEE?"

"Yes! Amy here," I say, tossing my two-year old *Maclean's* magazine back on a stack, then following the technician down the hall. She leads us both into a dark ultrasound room and points to a reclining chair. "Please seat yourself," she murmurs.

The chair is high, so I slide from the edge to the middle, over an expanse of waxy sanitary paper, crumpling and apologizing as I go.

We sit in awkward silence—me on the ruffled paper, Josh on a wheeled chair beside me, the technician in front of the ultrasound machine. The stillness is broken only by a soft hum from the computers, the clatter of the technician's typing, and the crinkle of me nervously shifting my weight.

"According to your file," the technician says, "you are eight weeks pregnant. We will listen for a heartbeat, but if we don't find one, we won't be alarmed. It is still quite early in the pregnancy. Have you drunk thirty-two ounces of water in the last hour and a half?

"I have," I say, rather proudly.

"Good. A full bladder helps us get a clear picture. Now—please bare your stomach."

I modestly uncover a few inches of my stomach, but the technician spreads my clothes further, leaving a wide swath of skin. I feel exposed, naked even, as I survey my flat, pale stomach glowing in the blue light of the computer monitors. My freckles are dark, like speckles of black ink, and my lower ribs protrude as I nervously suck in my breath.

"You can watch up there," the technician says, pointing high on the wall where a flat screen crackles to life with a vague scene resembling a snowstorm in car headlights.

She spreads gel over an ultrasound wand and then, with a single word of warning—"cold," presses the iciness against my belly-button. As the technician inches the wand one direction and then another, a dark patch forms on the screen above us. In its centre is a simple orb, like a tiny pearl in an oyster shell.

"The dark patch is the sac surrounding the embryo," the technician explains. "The circle in the middle is the embryo. The entire embryo is approximately a half inch long. Your baby's lungs are forming and the brain is developing. Arms and legs are present even if they are too small to see."

She freezes the screen and hits the zoom function, quadrupling the pearl's size. The pearl throbs and then a scratchy thump begins. The technician adjusts the speaker volume until the thumping becomes a triumphant drumbeat: Ba bum, ba bum, ba bum.

"The heart is nice and strong," she says. "Ninety-five beats per minute, typical for this stage."

"Beautiful," I whisper.

Josh and I gaze wide-eyed at the throbbing orb. To glimpse inside yourself and watch some part of you function is remarkable enough, but to peer at the beginning of a human life—this is truly miraculous.

The technician slides the wand away from the sounds of the baby's heartbeat toward the perimeter of the screen, freezing the view to take measurements. "Cervix...uterus...it all looks good," she says.

After ten minutes of picture taking, she powers off the machine and hands me a stiff paper towel to dry my stomach. "I'll forward the results to your doctor, and if there is cause for concern you'll hear from her. For now, you are free to go. The washroom is in the hall."

I had forgotten how badly I need the washroom, mesmerized as I was by the magic of the ultrasound. But as I stand in the tiny room, hovering over the sink, wondering whether to sit on the toilet or throw up in it, I breathe a sigh of relief. Everything is okay.

• • •

I SPEND CHRISTMAS ON THE COUCH, EATING CHINESE TAKEOUT while we make Skype calls to our parents. We treat ourselves to a weekend in Toronto—"Nutcracker" at the National Ballet, steak dinners, a hotel with an outdoor winter pool—but I'm sick the whole time and we're caught in two blizzards, one while we crunch down Yonge Street, the other while we fight our way home on the 401. By the time we return to find a foot of snow on our driveway, we're almost sorry we left.

January and February inch by and we yearn for spring, or at least for the days to lengthen out of their wintry gloom.

By Valentine's Day, I'm eighteen weeks pregnant and twenty pounds heavier. I worry I'll balloon to the size of a bulldozer, never again a size six. Josh paints the nursery and I order furniture, white and light, perfect for a baby. We read the pregnancy guides and register for a group prenatal class on labour and delivery. We pore over a book on baby names, marvelling at the modern monikers—Griffin, Cinsere, McKaty. We price-compare strollers, car seats, high chairs and swings. We book our summer holidays and put our finances in order. By the time we see our baby's delicate face on the twenty-week ultrasound in early March, we're prepared.

Chapter 3

IT'S A WEDNESDAY MORNING IN THE MIDDLE OF MARCH, ALREADY 10 o'clock by the time I roll out of bed. I pause at the full-length mirror to muse upon the absurdity of my reflection. I'm wearing pyjamas, pink verging on Hollywood cerise. The top stretches over my pregnant stomach like a gunny sack stuffed with a cantaloupe. The pants' elastic band settles somewhere below my waist line. My eyes are tired, my pale face puffy. I look less than my five feet, four inches, slouched as I am against the bed.

I yawn lazily at my reflection and wonder if I have anything clean to wear. I've outgrown my regular clothes and don't have many maternity clothes. They're expensive, especially considering they're only required for a few months, and are mostly designed along the lines of cadet pup tents. If I wanted a pup tent, I could run down to the local Army and Navy and see what's in stock. It would certainly save money.

I have searched for attractive maternity clothes. For weeks and weeks, I've browsed endless online images of cheerful, thin-faced models with fake bumps beckoning me to add garments to my virtual cart and click through to exorbitant shipping charges, but despite my best efforts I come up empty.

"Right, and how does that not look like a tent dress?" I mutter as Josh, ever patient, justifies the shapelessness.

"You have to wear something," he says. "Everyone knows you're pregnant, so what's the big deal? You might as well be comfortable."

But this morning, it feels unnecessary to get dressed at all. I'm on March break from teaching, so I can be as lazy as I like.

I go downstairs. Breakfast. Emails. Studio work. Have I corrected Brooke's harmony homework? Did I order the Chopin Etudes for James?

I grab the latest issue of the *Clavier Companion* and head to the washroom. As I sit, reading an article on teaching compound metre to young children, I feel something strange, deep inside of me. Like a balloon being blown up, a pressure grows, filling space that shouldn't be filled. Puzzled, I push against the pressure I feel inside of me and the ballooning sensation returns. I stand up and look down.

The toilet is filled with blood. Blood drips down my legs, then splatters into the crimson pool forming around feet. I reach down and am alarmed to feel something wet, like smashed grapefruit, protruding from my body. I pull my hand away and it's bloody too.

I stop breathing for a second, then grab the sink to stop the room from spinning. There has to be a reasonable explanation for the bleeding, but I can't think of it. My brain is moving too slowly. This can't be labour—I still have seventeen more weeks to go and I'm not in pain. But something is coming out of me, something soft and bloody. What is happening?

• • •

"WHY DIDN'T I CALL AN AMBULANCE?" I MUTTER TO MYSELF.

There's no parking at the hospital. Nothing. Lots A and B are full. There's no way to fit in one more car and everywhere I look there are restrictions: no parking at the curb, at a drop-off zone, in the ambulance corridor. I circle the hospital campus twice, blood and who-knows-what-else falling out of me, but the lots are all full. No room in the inn.

I briefly consider deserting the car on an ice-covered perennial bed, but I spy a coin-meter space on the opposite side of the street. There's barely enough room to park—vehicles cover the faint yellow pavement lines on both ends—but it's the only spot that's free. I turn the car around between towering snowbanks pushed up by snowploughs and return. As I put the car in reverse, my heart beats in a queer, quick staccato, throbbing as if there isn't quite enough room in my chest cavity. I wish Josh were with me, but he's in a cab somewhere, hurrying from work to meet me in Emergency.

I've never been very good at parallel parking, and on my first try I come in too sharp, my back right tire mounting the snow-covered curb, my front end still protruding into the street. I pull out and try again, and my second attempt is more promising. Even though I nudge the curb, I keep reversing until my bumper is inches from the Jeep behind me. The spot is tight, but it will do.

I don't have coins for the meter, but that doesn't feel important. Springing the car from impoundment may not be the biggest problem of the day. I power lock the car twice until the horn beeps, then pick my way over icy ruts, struggling to keep my balance.

Over the winter, snowploughs have skimmed the pavement, leaving behind a layer of snow which is polished into pure treachery. I step, then slide, then step again. Those of northern climates know this stiff-kneed hobble. Every limb braces for a swift and nearly certain crash to the ice below.

As I approach the entrance, a taxi pulls up at the curb and Josh jumps out. I squint into the sunshine, calling his name against the wail of an ambulance leaving. He turns and waves, then skids across the ice toward me.

"Are you okay?" he asks, taking my arm.

"I don't know," I sniff, wiping my tears with the back of my mitts.

"Okay, don't cry, Love," he says. "Just come."

He holds my hand, and together we scramble toward the automatic doors that slide open and closed beneath one of the most terrifying words in the English language. Lit up in bright red capitals, "EMERGENCY" hangs over our heads.

• • •

THE OPENING OF THE AUTOMATIC DOORS TRIGGERS A BLAST OF HOT AIR from a ceiling heater. Suddenly, I'm sweating under my wool scarf. My coat hangs heavy. I feel clammy. I stuff my mittens into my purse, then rummage through my wallet for my health card. I find it wedged between Sobeys and Costco loyalty cards. Under a grid of shiny "Ontario" holograms, my headshot stares back at me. I looked worried in the picture, even then.

The Emergency triage clerk is protected from infectious diseases and maniacs by a Plexiglas wall that runs from the desk up to the ceiling. There's a small opening for documents at counter-level and a smattering of holes for speaking higher up. A sign taped on the wall warns of a zero tolerance policy for aggressive behaviour.

The clerk types at a computer, an enormous thermos at her elbow. I wait for her to look up before I shout as non-aggressively as I can through the opening, "Obstetrical emergency?"

"Fourth floor," she shouts back. "Do you need a wheelchair?"

"No, I'm not in pain. Where are the elevators?"

"Follow the red feet." She snaps her attention back to her computer screen, her crimson nails clicking more loudly than before.

We set off down the hall, following the red feet painted on the floor. On one side of the hall, an old man lies on a gurney. His legs are scarcely covered by a wrinkled sheet and his grey feet dangle off the thin mattress. He clasps a pillow over his ears, but I can still see spider veins stretching across his bald head. Beside him, a maintenance man perches on a ladder, precariously flicking about wires and tubing. His tool belt radio roars a reminder that yes, indeed, CFRA is Ottawa's only live, 24/7 talk radio station.

As the red feet turn to the left, the hallway narrows, and a sign marked "Short Term Care" hangs over the doorway. I look doubtfully from the sign to the people that line the hallway on straight-backed chairs like mourners at a wake.

"Josh, this can't be right!" I stop. "We're going into a ward, not toward an elevator."

"She said red feet," Josh says, pulling my hand and walking on.

At the end of the continually narrowing hallway, the red feet point to a heavy steel-hinged door, significant enough to be an entrance to another wing of the hospital. I shove it open, but immediately realize my mistake. Inside, an elderly woman lies on a gurney in what looks to be a supply room. She's naked, except for a single sheet that slides to the floor, and she mumbles incoherently, rocking back and forth in the fetal position.

I jump back, horrified. "Josh! I told you this was wrong."

We retrace our steps until we find a woman wearing a staff tag. She points to a set of unmarked doors and gives directions to the elevators with a shrug, as if any person with half a brain could find the elevators if they only applied themselves. We thank her, then push through the doors. Across a rotunda, elevator doors beep open.

"Hold, please!" Josh calls.

We squeeze into the elevator beside a geriatric patient nearly blocking the doorway with his electric wheelchair, a FedEx driver yelling into a cellphone—"Sorry! I'm going to lose you! I just got into an elevator"—and a pregnant young woman scolding the toddler in her arms—"You can't push the buttons. Stop fussing."

The elevator starts to climb and, at the fourth-floor chime, the doors open to a sign with "Obstetrical" as the lead adjective for every unit. Finally, we're in the right place.

Chapter 4

AT A DESK MARKED OBSTETRICAL ASSESSMENT UNIT, I SLIDE MY health card across the counter and say in a shaky voice, "I'm at twenty-three weeks and I'm bleeding rather badly."

With an unimpressed look, the clerk takes my card (I suppose I'm not the first of my kind), swipes it through a long slot on her keyboard, then frowns.

"I don't see any record of you in the hospital database," she says. "You need to go to Maternity admissions, register, and then come back here."

"Really?" I sputter. "I don't know that I need to be admitted. I just need to get checked out."

"Really." Her voice is flat and humourless.

I pause, forming yet another protestation, but Josh steers my shoulders toward the Maternity admissions desk. "There's no point arguing, Amy. It just slows things down."

I know arguing is futile, but I still smart at the bureaucratic insensitivity. I could be losing my baby, but I still need to be swiped into the system. Surely that can be dealt with later. It's not that I don't have a health card. I just showed it!

The young woman at the second desk hardly glances up as we approach.

"Hi," I say curtly. "Triage told me I need to register here, then go back."

"Health card?"

I hand it to her, and she slowly copies my name and address onto the electronic form on her screen. She tilts her head to read what she's typed, her mouth open, pink gum circulating. After a little more reading and a little more typing, she repeatedly whacks the backspace key: TAP-TAP-TAP-TAP-TAP. I suspect we are making no progress at all.

"Okay, like, I'm gonna need you to, like, confirm the stuff on your card," she intones in that annoying voice, popularized by pubescent hair stylists filming YouTube tutorials.

I rattle off my address and she nods, painfully slowly. "Awesome. Your mother's maiden name?"

"S-S-Smith." I am crying now—there is no hope for it—but the girl at the computer never glances up. I'm just another patient losing her mind.

"Father's middle name?"

I draw a blank. I can't think. My dad goes by Don, but that isn't his first name. It's his second. What is she cross-referencing? Will Robert, his actual first name, but not the name he uses, come up as his second name? I'm stuck, tongue-tied, but then I realize she probably isn't cross-referencing anything, just creating a profile. I could say "Howard" and it would make no difference.

"Donald," I sniff, scanning the hallway, desperate for someone to help me though the madness. To my surprise, I spot Dr. Vincent, my obstetrician, wearing a surgical cap, pushing a patient into a recovery room down the hall. Our eyes meet and her mouth opens in a silent inquiry. Concern wrinkles her brow.

Thank God! I think. She will come. She will sort things out for me.

"So, like, take this form down to Triage"—the girl slides a clipboard across the counter—"and have a nice day."

Have a "nice day"? What is this girl thinking? I'm checking into a Labour and Delivery ward at twenty-three weeks! How many women have nice days after doing that? I want to say as much to the girl, whose biggest goal in life seems to be maintaining a spray-bottle tan and exasperating pregnant Ottawa women, but I don't say anything, not even a "thank you." I just walk away and Josh follows.

The obstetrical assessment unit clerk casts a quick eye over the clipboard, then whisks us into a small room behind her counter.

"Take off your clothes, waist down, and sit on the observation chair," she says. "You can cover up with this." She hands me a stiff flannel sheet that has been washed too many times in the powerful hospital detergent that eradicates all germs, bacteria and comfort, then pulls a blue curtain around us, leaving me to undress in privacy.

I feel the draft of the March morning creep through the vertical window blinds as I take off my clothes, one layer at time. The floor tiles feel icy, so I stand on tiptoes as Josh wraps the sheet around me.

"I'm sure it's nothing," I say with false bravado as I hoist myself up onto the observation chair.

Josh gathers my clothes into a tight bundle and smiles, but his smile is unconvincing. We're both upset and there's little point pretending otherwise.

"Is there much blood?" I ask, embarrassed.

"Some," Josh says, folding my clothes carefully to hide the stains. He stacks my clothes onto the wide windowsill, then sits beside me, holding my hand. Together we wait. It's impossible to say for how long; time passes at an odd pace when your mind is racing.

After a while, a nurse enters, pushing back the curtain. She carries a pencil and my clipboard, and she wears a surgical cap as if she's been pulled from a C-section to deal with me.

"I'm going to ask you a few questions before the resident examines you," she says. "Let's start with age."

"Twenty-seven."

"First pregnancy?"

"Yes."

"How far along are you?"

"Twenty-three weeks plus one day."

"Any difficulty before?"

"Some bleeding at six to eight weeks."

"Nothing since then?"

"No."

The nurse scribbles notes, then proceeds in a calm voice I suppose is most commonly used by police psychologists talking jumpers down from bridges: "Drug use?"

"No."

"Alcohol?"

"No."

"Previous miscarriages, still births, or terminated pregnancies?"

"No."

"And what happened this morning?"

"I was using the washroom and I felt pressure as if a balloon was blowing up inside of me. The toilet was filled with blood and I could feel something protruding."

Her head whips up from the chart. "Something protruding?"

"Yes. Like smashed flesh."

She stares at me for a second, then shudders, almost imperceptibly.

"I'll be right back," she says, dashing from the room, letting the door bang behind her.

Her response worries me.

"Everything is going to be okay, don't you think?" I ask Josh. "This sort of thing happens all the time and babies still survive, don't they? I think so. I'm pretty sure they do."

I talk to calm my nerves, hoping to gain assurance by saying what I want to be true, but Josh calmly rubs my cold fingers in his warm palm. "We just have to see, Babe," he says.

"I know."

"Relax, okay? Don't add anxiety to the equation."

I lie back and look around. The triage room (or "patient environment," as fundraisers are apt to call them) is simply furnished. Beyond the observation chair, a stainless steel sink, and a few wall-mounted cabinets, it's empty. Sterile and colourless, it's a purgatory for the expectant. Admission to a labour room or discharge to rutted ice and a parking ticket? That is the question.

The nurse with the surgical cap returns with a resident who looks about my age. Indian or Sri Lankan perhaps, she's dressed in the universal blue scrubs of the Ottawa Hospital. Her spiral-curly hair is wound up in a high bun. She snaps on pale latex gloves, then wheels a stool to the foot of my observation chair.

"Hi, Amy," she says. "I'm sorry you're here today. We're going to check you out, okay?"

"Yep." I nod, hurriedly. I want to know what is happening to me.

"I need you to put your feet in the stirrups," she says, "and keep lying back as we lower you. You may feel the speculum as I take a look. Sorry, but it'll be cold."

The resident flips the sheet back over my knees and disappears from view as the nurse lowers the observation chair into a reclined position. I look up and make some joke about how cartoons on the ceiling would be a good idea, like at the dentist or blood clinic, but I don't make it to the punchline before the resident pulls the sheet over my legs and snaps off her gloves.

I'm confused though. I haven't felt anything, not her fingers, not the cold speculum, nothing. How can she be finished her assessment?

She tosses her gloves in the garbage, then sits beside me on the bed. Her eyes are glossy. She clears her throat.

"Look, Amy," she whispers, taking my hand. "I'm terribly sorry, but you have bulging membranes. I didn't even have to use the speculum; I can see them outside your body. You're probably completely dilated."

"What do you mean?"

"You will most likely deliver today." She stares hard at me.

"But it's too early!" I look frantically at Josh, willing him to correct her. Why is he crying? Why doesn't he tell her this can't happen right now?

"I know, I know, Sweetheart," the resident says, "but when you were using the toilet this morning, you were probably pushing the baby out."

"Why would the baby come out? I'm not in labour! It's way too early." I'm sobbing now.

"Sometimes these things happen and we don't know why."

"Is there anything you can do?" I say, as my chest heaves with half breaths.

The resident looks at the nurse and the nurse looks away. Neither one of them answers. Perhaps they don't want to say the thing I'm terrified of hearing.

Finally, the resident speaks: "I'm going to consult with Dr. Vincent—she's on call and she's your obstetrician anyway. We'll discuss a plan. Stay lying down. Don't move. If the baby is sliding out, we don't want to add gravity."

The resident flings back the blue curtain and disappears. I turn to the nurse who still stands in the middle of the room, perhaps wondering what to do next.

"Do babies survive at twenty-three weeks?" I whisper.

The nurse sucks her bottom lip for a second before kindly answering, "No. Not often. But Dr. Vincent will probably send you for an ultrasound to see if there's anything we can do."

"Like what? What can you do?"

"Sometimes we can do a cerclage to close the cervix. But I don't know if it would work for you. This is extremely early in the pregnancy to have membranes bulging outside the body. Some bulging can happen beyond the cervix, but bulging outside the body is a huge complication. The doctor might have a plan though." She shrugs optimistically, but I can see she doesn't believe what she's saying. She's thinks it's hopeless. I can tell.

Josh and I clutch hands. Life was normal when we woke, but now it's spinning out of control. We've always been blessed with excellent health and good fortune, but now we're losing our baby. In our families, old people die, but not babies. Babies are born healthy and grow up chubby. They don't die in a delivery room. This doesn't happen to us. But as much as I want to believe everything is a mistake, I know it isn't. I felt the pressure, the ballooning, the crushed flesh. There's still blood flowing out of me. I can't take comfort in denial.

Hurried footsteps pause outside the door. I hear Dr. Vincent whispering, "I just saw her the other day! She was in for her twenty-week appointment. She was fine!" and the resident insisting, "The membranes are bulging out. I can see them without a speculum."

The door opens and Dr. Vincent steps softly into the room like a funeral director easing in the casket. She looks as anxious as the resident, which does not comfort me. She pats my leg and I see tears in her eyes too. I wonder if everyone is crying.

"I'm so sorry to see you here, Amy," she whispers. "This is entirely unexpected and you didn't do anything to cause this. These things happen. We're going to do an ultrasound and, once we see what's going on, we'll determine if anything can be done."

"The nurse mentioned sewing me up," I say.

"Yes, a cerclage. I'm not sure that would work because I suspect the membranes are too far extended. But we'll see. For now, I have a stretcher in the hallway. We'll lift you on it and wheel you down to Ultrasound. I don't want you sitting or standing from now on."

I relax my body so the nurses can easily roll me onto one side then the other as they spread a cool sheet beneath me. Three of them take corners of the sheet with Josh on the fourth and, after a quick countdown, they hoist me onto the stretcher. Someone tucks a pillow under my head and, from then on, my view is restricted to the ceiling and a few feet of wall.

They push me quickly down the hall, toward the ultrasound unit, but it's all surreal. I feel panicked and the medical team looks worried, yet all around us hospital floors are being washed; food trays, carried; congratulatory flowers, delivered. Strangers are unconcerned. They don't stand aside with hands raised in gestures of good will. They squeeze past as if our mere existence inconveniences them.

When the nurses stop the stretcher, I raise my head to see a hallway lined with expectant mothers guzzling from water bottles and rubbing their backs. Some have impatient husbands and small children with them. All have big stomachs and they stare curiously at my relatively flat one.

"I can take her here!" someone calls and the nurses push me into an ultrasound room. The door is closed and the room is dark, but it doesn't feel cozy like on earlier visits. Little green machine lights flicker like winking cats. Fans growl. Monitors cast odd blue shadows over my white hands. I stare up at gloomy corners as Dr. Vincent whispers to the ultrasound technician, "She's at twenty-three weeks and has severely bulging membranes. We need to know if there is any chance of a cerclage, so try to get detailed pictures of the cervix. We also need the baby's fetal heart rate."

Dr. Vincent disappears to the hall, and the technician pats my arm. "Do you want the monitor shut off?" she gently asks.

"No, I want to see," I say, pulling the sheet off my stomach so she can begin.

The technician covers the ultrasound wand with gel, then presses it to my stomach as the ceiling monitor flickers to life with grainy shadows. To my untrained eye, the flecks of muscles and tissues seem to be holding together in a tight, protective sac, but the technician takes measurements—digital white lines in frozen screen shots—with a frown on her face. The miniscule dashes and slashes measure distances between bits of me I'll never actually see, chunks of anatomy I never thought would fail. The technician recognizes the abnormalities, but I don't. I just wait, breath held, eyes burning, until she finally moves the wand up my stomach and a tiny body comes into view on the screen above our heads. The arms waves and the feet kick. The movements synchronize with the movements I feel inside of me. Then, with wide, sweeping gestures, the baby turns to face the ultrasound wand.

A stubby nose. Closed eyes. A pretty mouth. The angelic little face shreds any composure I have left. My nerves aren't strong enough to stand all that innocent beauty dangling between life and death.

I cover my face with my trembling hands and rock back and forth while Josh wraps his arm around my head and whispers something I don't hear. The technician lays down the wand, and the baby's face slips away. And that's it. We've said goodbye.

Chapter 5

DR. VINCENT HAS THAT AWFUL LOOK ON HER FACE. THE DESPER-
ately kind one that doctors use when they have to tell you horrible
things.

"There's nothing we can do," she says. "The cervix can't be sewn
shut because it doesn't exist anymore. Normally, it meets like this"—
she holds her hands together, finger nails touching—"but for some
reason yours has totally opened, and the membranes have essentially
fallen out"—she pulls her fingers back, leaving a gap of air.

"There's nothing you can do?" Josh asks with disbelief in his voice.

"I'm so sorry. Amy will stay in hospital until the baby is born.
It might be today, or tomorrow, or a week from now. I don't know.
Anything could happen."

I wipe tears and mascara from my stinging eyes. "But what if the
baby is born today?" I choke.

"A neonatologist will explain your options. You are at twenty-three
weeks and, though it's possible for your baby to survive, it's not very
likely. The best-case scenario is that you lie here for as long as you
can. If you can get to twenty-four or twenty-five weeks, there might
be a chance of survival but right now the odds are not very good."

"Do you think the baby will come right away?"

"Anything is possible, but in my experience I'd say—yes. The baby
will likely come before the end of the day."

I cover my eyes. This can't be happening. This is what it feels like
to lose a child. The shock. The loss. The gut-punching realization
that life can end in a second, and dreams can vanish like they never
existed at all.

"I know it's a lot to absorb, but we're here to help," Dr. Vincent
soothes. "Let's get you into a Labour and Delivery room and we'll go
from there."

I'm pushed back out into the hallway lit by a dozen heartless fluorescents. I'm too miserable to care who sees me crying now. I let my tears flow as the ceiling passes above me both at the speed of lightning and in slow motion. I know that no matter what happens next, life will never be the same. This is going to change everything, whatever this is.

I'm headed to Labour and Delivery, but I'm not ready to labour or deliver. I haven't earned the right. I'm cheating on this pregnancy thing and I'm going to get caught at it. How can a baby born seventeen weeks early survive?

I'm still crying when the bed brakes click on and a strong hand takes mine. I open my eyes to see a nurse hovering over me. Her face is lined. Her thick, charcoal hair is piled on top of her head like a Sikh's turban. Her stocky frame strains even the shapelessness of her hospital-issued blue scrubs. She exudes strength, and an image of the magnificent eighteenth–century Russian empress Catherine the Great comes to mind.

"I'm Janice, your nurse," she says firmly, breaking through my fog. "I know you've had terrible news, but we're going to do everything we can to keep this baby inside."

She hands me a tissue to wipe my face, and I have a feeling that crying is over for the moment.

"Now," Janice says, her hands on her hips, "I've paged Dr. Shumar to come and discuss options with you. He is a senior neonatologist and has been with us for twenty years at least. You'll be in good hands. Until then, Josh has gone down to Admissions to finish up your paper work and I've had instructions to put you in the Trendelenburg position."

"What's that?" I ask, sniffing.

Janice hits a lever on the bed and, ever so slowly, my head and shoulders tilt downwards. By the time she nods in satisfaction, I'm looking at the intersection of the wall and ceiling tiles above me. My head pounds with the extra flow of blood though I'm probably only tilted ten degrees toward the floor.

"That is Trendelenburg," Janice says. "Named after a German surgeon from back in the day. The idea is that gravity helps keep the baby inside if your head is lower than your feet. Not pleasant, I know. It feels like you're standing on your head."

"And I stay like this?" I ask, swallowing hard as something akin to claustrophobia sweeps over me.

"For as long as you can."

"But what about the bathroom?"

"That's the next step." Janice rummages through a cart of medical supplies, pulling out what looks like a long thread and a needle. "You're going to be catheterized."

I gasp. "Will it hurt?"

"Mostly likely." Janice retrieves a heavy plastic drainage bag and some antiseptic wipes from the cart, then unravels the blood-stained sheets from around my legs. "Close your eyes and think of something pleasant."

I close my eyes and suck in my breath, but I can't think of one pleasant thing. It's all too horrible.

Janice counts down—"3. 2. 1."—as a pain, sharp and quick, stabs through my groin. It feels like a flash of fire, then a burn.

"It's all right. I'm done." Janice fastens a piece of tape around the catheter line, then covers me with a fresh sheet. "You'll get used to it. Next, I'll connect an IV. The jury is still out among researchers whether or not hydration keeps contractions at bay, but we'll err on the side of safety and get a saline solution going. Can't do any harm."

From my limited viewpoint, I see Janice retrieving an IV pole from a storage cupboard, and a bag of saline solution and a needle from her commodious cart. She ties an elastic tourniquet around my upper arm and thumbs the inside of my right elbow. She squints, then aligns a needle with a small mauve vein in my arm. I close my eyes and hold my breath, but the IV needle is less painful than the catheter needle so I breathe again.

"There you go," Janice says, tidying up her supplies. "Nothing to do now but wait. You might not have the baby for days or even weeks. I'll leave so the neonatologist can come for counselling."

• • •

DR. SHUMAR WASTES NO TIME. A SHORT MAN IN A LAB COAT AND necktie, he's no sooner in the room than he begins talking, quickly and efficiently. He chooses his words carefully, favouring precise medical terms over more common expressions: fetus over baby; prognosis over guess; mortality over death.

"This is not an optimal situation," he says, stating the obvious, "but we are here to help you through this difficult time. I pulled up your previous ultrasound image and the one from this morning. I see no correlation. Hmmm? Nothing on the ultrasound from several weeks ago indicated that the cervix was opening. Unfortunately, these things happen and we don't know why. There is no reason to feel guilt or remorse."

I nod my head. I hadn't felt guilt or remorse but I begin to consider both, now I know I shouldn't.

"From what I see today," the doctor goes on, "the membranes are bulging five to six centimetres beyond the cervix, which is completely dilated. In other words, there is nothing keeping the fetus from coming. Hmmm? So, what do we do? Number one, we keep you hydrated. Some research indicates that proper hydration holds off contractions. Number two, we keep you on bed rest with your head lower than your feet. Let gravity help. But these measures are not going to circumvent a preterm birth. You will give birth early. In preparation, we need to make an agreeable plan so that everyone— Mom, Dad, the medical staff—act as a team. Hmmm?"

"Of course," Josh murmurs, but I can't say anything. There is a massive glob of tears at the back of my throat.

Dr. Shumar opens a thick red folder and hands Josh a stack of papers.

"These are the average outcomes for extremely premature births in Ottawa," he says. "The numbers aren't perfect—many things influence outcomes. But in an otherwise normal pregnancy like yours, a baby born at twenty-three weeks gestation will have less than a ten-percent chance of surviving without extreme physical or developmental disabilities."

He pauses, allowing us time to absorb that horrendous statistic.

"What percentage survives at all?" Josh asks in a shaky voice, eyeing me to see how I'm handling the conversation. I stare back at him, knowing we're both going to be crying soon.

"Less than thirty percent," the doctor replies flatly.

"And most of them have long-term disabilities?"

"Unfortunately, yes."

"What kinds of disabilities?" I ask.

"Well, cerebral palsy or neurological damage is most typical. Also, the lungs are not completely formed at twenty-three weeks, so even if we are able to resuscitate the baby and keep him or her alive, there are always serious concerns for the lungs' short-term and long-term function. Sometimes, at this early stage, the heart is not beating at birth. The question then becomes, do we apply compressions in an attempt to start the heart?"

"Do compressions work?" Josh asks.

"I do not recommend them. The force required to start the heart is enough to crush the chest and induce mortality. So why induce the trauma? Hmmm? It's senseless."

"So what should we do?" I ask.

"I cannot recommend one plan over another. In this hospital, we can only provide 'comfort care' for a baby that is born seventeen weeks premature. The baby is kept warm, given a sedative for pain, and is allowed to pass quietly in your arms."

I catch a sob at the back of my throat.

"I know. This is difficult." Dr. Shumar looks down, perhaps embarrassed by my display of emotion. "At twenty-three weeks, the situation is grave. If you still haven't given birth by twenty-three weeks plus five days, then maybe we can transfer you to the Grace Hospital where they have the equipment to resuscitate the smallest of babies. But you must know, a transfer will be risky. If you go into labour on the way, the paramedics will not be able to save your baby. But if you make it to the Grace and give birth around twenty-four weeks, the odds of the baby's survival increase slightly."

"How much better are the odds at twenty-four weeks?" Josh asks.

"You are looking at a sixty-percent chance of survival. Out of that, a third will have dramatic disabilities, a third will be mildly disabled, and a third will experience normal health. In your case, lung function would also improve because we'd have time to administer a steroid injection for the baby's lungs."

I look at Josh, hoping for some brave insight, but he just looks stunned.

"So maybe we need to stay here for a few days?" I offer tentatively, not knowing if what I'm suggesting is medically or even ethically appropriate. "Maybe I should rest until we get closer to twenty-four weeks. Then, as the odds of survival improve, we could risk the transfer. What do you think, Doctor?"

"As I said, I cannot recommend one path over another and I don't need an answer right now. You can think over things. Transferring is risky, yes, but we can't offer the treatment you'll need here at this hospital. However, even at the Grace, it still might be too early for a successful resuscitation."

He pauses as the paging system crackles from the hallway, "Calling Dr. Shumar to Triage. Dr. Shumar to Triage."

"I must go, but I will remain in contact throughout the day in case labour begins."

As he leaves, we politely thank him for his time as if he's a life insurance salesman we're anxious to be rid of, even if he does warn us of inevitability. Somehow, we still want to believe these decisions don't have to be made.

Josh moves close to me. His eyes are red and the hair along his temples is tousled from him grabbing at it. He lays his head on my chest and his hot tears trickle over my neck, soaking my nightgown. His breath is warm and I stroke his shoulder.

"Oh, Josh. What are we going to do?" I whisper, but he doesn't answer.

The facts are ghastly and no solution is obvious. Even the best-case scenario—lying in a hospital bed for a few weeks with my feet in the air waiting to give birth to a micro preemie with little chance of survival—seems appalling. And that's the best-case scenario. Several other scenarios vie for worst-case scenario, but I try not to think about them.

"This is such a shock," I whisper.

"Disasters usually are."

"So, what are we going to do?" I ask again, but with less expectation of an answer.

I know people who have lost babies, but they talk calmly about the loss, with detachment and poise. I can't fathom delivering a stillborn baby or holding a baby as it dies. That kind of bravery exists outside my small sack of talents. I have no resources for coping in the face of death, no lessons learned from prior adversities. I live in Canada, not a Third World country, and I cling to the innocent belief that death can always be put off until another day, that some miraculous procedure is always available.

We lie quietly, me on the delivery bed, Josh as close as he can manage. Our thoughts hover above the gritty details of hospital life. While tests are ordered and paper work is filed, we contemplate life and death. Suddenly, we are evaluating all our convictions. How far should we go to save our baby's potentially unviable life? No one has the correct answer; they just have options. Data. Percentages. They expect us to make decisions based on our own beliefs, but everything I've believed since childhood about the sanctity of life seems irrelevant. I was taught that life should be saved at all stages, without exception. No matter the risks, every life should be fought for. But now I don't know what I believe. Just because we might be able to keep the baby alive, does that mean we should? What if the little one suffers horribly because of our decision?

Despite these moral abstractions, we must consider tangible things. The car is still parked at an empty coin meter, and Josh's cellphone is chirping a text message alert nearly constantly.

With a sigh, Josh pulls his head off my chest and thumbs through his messages. Our parents are inquiring, he says. They want answers too. He punches out a text message, then reaches for his coat.

"I'm going to move the car into a parking lot," he murmurs, stroking my hand. "I'll be back as quickly as I can."

• • •

NURSE JANICE TAKES A CHAIR, CROSSING HER LEGS WITH A SIGH. "So you've decided to stay here for a day or two, then transfer?"

"Do you think that's a good decision?" I ask, already knowing how she'll answer.

"No one can tell you what is or isn't a good decision," she predictably replies. "I think it's wise to rest here for a bit so we can get you stable. We wouldn't want you to go into labour on the Queensway, yet there's very little we can do for you here. You have to trust your instincts, because there is no right or wrong. Even the doctors don't know what's best."

"Have women lasted for weeks in these situations?"

"Goodness, yes! I remember a woman, fifteen years ago, who lay in hospital from week twenty to twenty-nine. She gave birth to a healthy baby; small, yes, but healthy."

"Did she lose her mind?"

"I'm sure she thought she would, but it was her backache that nearly drove her round the bend."

"I can believe that," I mutter.

"But it is possible to extend the pregnancy through bed rest, and it is for the best. If you can lie quietly for a week, two weeks even, it will make all the difference to your baby's outcome. Even a day or two is useful."

I nod, struggling to understand what is required of me. It seems that I just need to "be." Nothing more. All my activities are now condensed to the simple verb "be." Exist. Stay still. Relax. Don't upset yourself. Don't get up. Don't dress. Don't do anything. Make no effort of any kind. Just survive one rotation of the clock into another, hour after hour, day after day, until the baby arrives. It's an unusual alignment of priorities. It's like a massive set of brakes grinding my body to a halt. It's almost laughable, it's so odd.

"You'll get used to this, Honey. It's all been so sudden," Janice soothes, as if she can read my mind, then she goes on more cheerfully, explaining meal schedules and shift changes, introducing me to the workings of the institution within which I'll spend the foreseeable future. She chats easily, but the more I listen, the more uneasy I feel. Janice is moving me into a new normal. Hospital routines and dire statistics are now my points of reference. I am immersed in the realities and maintenance of the disaster.

Eventually, she leaves and I'm alone for the first time since rushing to the hospital. My adrenaline evaporates. My energy vanishes. I close my eyes against the dim, late-afternoon light that fogs the room in grainy shadows. Already, the peculiar smells of disinfectant and detergent are becoming less pungent, more familiar. The intercoms catch less and less of my attention; their scratchy pleas for personnel to dash one way or another are less urgent to my ear. Little by little, my anxious thoughts dissolve into puffs of sadness and then cease to be thoughts at all.

Chapter 6

SUPPER CARTS RATTLE SOMEWHERE OUTSIDE MY ROOM. I OPEN MY eyes, but I don't see a food tray. Maybe it hasn't got here yet.

I rub my tired eyes with my left hand. My right hand has an IV line taped to it, so I leave it lying limply beside me. I've only been on bed rest for six hours, but my back is already throbbing. I probably have an exaggerated sense of the pain with so little to think about, just the trauma of the day to brood over.

Josh dozes in a reclining chair beside me, snoring slightly. His head lolls over his left shoulder, exposing his white, razor-rubbed jaw. His legs sprawl awkwardly in front of him. Every time he shifts his weight, the PVC upholstery makes strange rubbing noises.

I glare at the wall clock, my ears pricking with each tick. Seconds pass so slowly that I wonder if something is wrong with the clock. It's like I'm eight years old again, jammed in the back seat between two older sisters on a road trip to the mountains, being told to sit still. As it is, I can't shift one way or another even if I want to. My body weighs down my head, ploughing my shoulders into the mattress. I keep thinking horrible things, over and over—things about the baby, things about my body, things about a future I can't rationalize away. I'm stuck, in every sense of the word.

The door opens and an overhead light flicks on. The beam shines straight into my eyes so I turn my head sharply to avoid it. Undoubtedly, the light was intended to aid surgery, not bask a patient in a gentle glow.

"Supper tray!" a uniformed lad chirps as he hurries into the room, whizzes a tray onto a counter, then disappears. Labour and Delivery is probably not a favourite ward for young, male kitchen porters.

"Josh, darling," I murmur. "Would you shut off that light?"

Josh opens his eyes, one at a time, curls his shoulders into a stretch and yawns. The stress of the day has taken its toll on him too. He looks exhausted, yet he is instantly caring. "Did you sleep a bit?" he asks. "Are you in any pain? Can I get you anything?"

He's such a marvel, my husband. His kindness and gentleness are what attracted me to him in the first place. I remember the Christmas I brought him home to meet my family. He read my young nieces and nephews through an eight-inch stack of Berenstain Bears twice, doing the voices, never skipping the boring bits. In the space of a holiday season, I decided there was a lot of good in a guy who would do that.

I watch him shuffle over to the light switch in search of a softer light, his dress shirt untucked, its wrinkled tails hanging over his suit pants. He adjusts the lighting, then lifts the cover on the food tray (no steam cloud emerges) and looms over the meal quizzically, as if he's opened a hand-knitted pullover as a birthday present and is formulating a polite response.

"I'm not a hundred percent certain," he says, "but it could be chicken and rice. Should I feed you some?"

"Yes, I guess, though it may be tricky with my head so low."

Josh sets the tray on the over-bed table and cranks the whiny lift until the table is high enough to fit over my legs. He pushes it over my chest, then sits close beside me. With an encouraging smile, he drops a spoonful of the chicken concoction into my mouth.

Being fed when I'm not sick makes me feel infantile, but I have to accept the help, lying as I am with my head below my feet. The position isn't conducive to swallowing either. The chicken rebels against descending, bobbing and swirling at the back of my throat. I attempt to catch a drop of sauce with my tongue, but it rolls onto the pillow.

Josh rips a thin paper napkin out of its plastic wrap and waves away my apologies. "Don't worry; I've got it," he says, dabbing the spot clean. "Supper up to snuff?"

"I had a worse meal on a red-eye to Taiwan once, but only just. I think they cooked the chicken down to mush for the geriatric patients who didn't make it to the hospital with their teeth."

Josh loads the spoon again. "There is one piece of good news from this afternoon. The car wasn't towed; however, there was a $100 ticket on it."

"To be expected. I didn't have coins, maybe a quarter, and that wasn't going to solve any problems. At least it wasn't towed."

"Also, I went home and got you some stuff: toothpaste, a sweater, that sort of thing. Open your mouth, Love." He drops in some more chicken.

"Are you going to spend the night?" I mumble hopefully.

"Of course. I wouldn't leave you alone."

Josh munches on a dry bread roll (also packaged in plastic), and pours a bit of water into a flimsy cup for us to share. It's an impromptu picnic, but we aren't enjoying a pastoral revel on chartreuse grass with refreshing breezes. Instead, as the daylight fades, we glumly listen to an ambulance siren rising and falling with the gusts of wind that slam against the window. The siren makes me think of lying in bed at night as a child, listening to the coyotes, their howls driving our own civilized farm dog to distraction. There isn't a lonelier sound in the world than coyotes howling, except maybe an ambulance siren, fading into the night.

"I think I'm moving through the stages of grief," I say, breaking the silence. "I'm over the shock and am headlong into anger. Everything was going fine, then this. It's so disappointing."

Josh stares unblinkingly out the dark window. His jaw clamps shut and his brown eyes swim. I wonder how many tears he cried this afternoon while I panicked. Yes, it was my body everyone rushed around—scanning, needling, patting—but it is also his child causing the uproar. I'm the transportation, the train compartment in which our little one is chugging into this world, but he owns the chaos as much as I do. The only difference is that he has the use of his legs whereas I will become more familiar with the crooked ceiling panels hanging over my head.

• • •

"ARE YOU BLEEDING MUCH?"

It's nearly night and Nurse Janice has come to change my IV bag. She unhooks the used, wrinkled bag from its pole and attaches a plump new one.

"I can't feel anything," I say, helplessly.

"I'll check." Janice flips the sheets back from my legs and draws a sharp breath. "Oh, Amy!" she exclaims. "You're badly bleeding. We'll have to change the sheets."

"I'm sorry," I whisper. "I couldn't tell."

It feels like another chink in my armour of dignity, not that there is anything dignified about childbirth anyway. Exposure is inevitable and might as well be accepted—unabashedly, unapologetically.

"Don't be sorry," Janice says. "I've seen blood. It's a Maternity ward, after all."

She bangs a cupboard door and must find fresh bedding for she and Josh gently lift my legs and slide a smooth, cool sheet under me. Her arms are as strong and steady as his, which I find surprising for a woman her age.

Josh bundles the stained sheets into a laundry hamper and, through the hamper's transparent blue bag, I see blood stains the colour of hamburger after thirty seconds in a frying pan.

"Why the bleeding, Janice?" I ask.

"It's hard to say. According to the ultrasound, your membranes aren't ruptured, just damaged, so they could be acting like an open sore, constantly oozing. Who knows? They may bleed until the baby is born. And remember: a little blood goes a long way and always looks nasty."

Janice settles me on a massive pad the size of a hand towel. It seems capable of absorbing all the blood in me. I know bleeding is to be expected during childbirth, but I've seen so much of my own blood today that I wonder if there is much left for when labour actually comes.

"Janice," I say softly, reaching out to touch her arm, "I was thinking, if I went into labour, like tonight, what would we do with the baby's body?"

"It depends on what you want. Some families want a burial, a service at the grave or something like that. In that case, the body is released to a funeral director who makes arrangements. Others families opt for cremation. You can take the ashes home."

I picture an urn on the mantelpiece and shudder.

"But don't worry, okay?" Janice pats my hand. "You don't have to decide what to do unless something happens."

I nod, tearing up, and Janice must sense my distress, for she moves on briskly: "I left some sheets for you, Josh," she says. "Just pull the handle under the chair and a bed will come popping out. Nothing to it. I know it's been a long day for you both, so try to get some sleep. That's what helps the most."

She wishes us a good night, then leaves, her NurseMates squeaking on the tiled floor, another twelve hours on tired feet finally over.

I wonder if she'll think of me when she sinks onto the couch beside her husband for the tail end of the hockey game. Will she say, "Had a bit of a sad one today," and will her husband reply, "These things happen," or will she even give me a second thought? Will I be filed away into her memory with forty years of other sad women, but barred from her private life, her everyday existence away from the hospital? "You got to leave it at the door. Can't take it home with you"—isn't that what experts say to people who have stressful jobs?

I don't know why it's important to me whether or not a complete stranger cares about me. I must be more traumatized than I understand to be concerned about that.

Chapter 7

SOMEONE ONCE SAID THAT THE WALLS OF HOSPITALS HEAR MORE prayers than the walls of churches, and it could well be true. The survival rate for the average church service is certainly better than that of many hospital wards, and there's nothing like facing mortality to turn one's thoughts to the immortal.

I pray during my first night in hospital. Again and again, I beg God for a normal full-term baby, even though I know my prayers won't be answered immediately. I'll have to wait. Waiting may be an inevitable aspect of life, a certainty even, but knowing that doesn't make it any easier. Instead, I lie awake and agonize over the unknown, over the events of the day which tumble together in my mind.

Josh sleeps soundly on the pullout chair beside me, but I watch the lights blinking on the machines around me and try not to think terrible thoughts—the baby is still alive, so everything could still turn out okay.

Eventually, I drift away, almost sleeping, but I can't stop my sub-conscious voices from whispering confusion. Maybe I'm at home, I think. Maybe I dreamed the nurses and the needles. Maybe none of this is real! I'm so certain I'm home in bed with Josh that I pat his firm, naked shoulder to prove it to myself. Of course, I whack the bed rail instead and wrench the IV needle in my hand. The pain wakes me and I'm disappointed. I had almost convinced myself I was dreaming.

Since childhood, I've sleepwalked and -talked. I've grown used to the fogginess between reality and my dream world. I know anything that seems real can actually be a figment of my overactive nocturnal imagination and, over time, my reaction has nearly become a double layer of dreaming: I acknowledge the dream, calm myself down, then press right on with it. "No, Amy," I might think, "you aren't naked on your wedding day. I don't care how many people are staring at you. It isn't possible that you forgot to dress. This is obviously a dream, so why don't you grab the tablecloth from the altar table and wrap it around yourself? That's right. The flannel one under the duvet."

Again and again, throughout the night, I drift off, then wake again, constantly confused why lights blink and intercoms scratch. In my more lucid moments, I yearn for even a hint of rising sun to glow through my window and end the misery of the lonely darkness. By morning, though, I'm a frantic Mrs. Rochester, locked away in the attic. I've been on bed rest for only eighteen hours and I'm already losing my grip.

• • •

"HELL-O-OH!" COOS THE MORNING NURSE CHEERFULLY.

"Please, Nurse," I beg, nearly in tears. "Can I roll onto my side for a bit? I'm in so much pain!"

"Call me Kathy. You need to avoid moving, but I can add a couple of towels under one side to tilt you."

"Please."

Nurse Kathy nudges me onto my left side, cramming a towel under my right. From this new position, I can see Josh sleeping on the chair-bed, legs curled, arms jammed against his chest.

"How's that?" she asks. "Comfy?"

"Better, thanks." I bite my lip and look away.

"Well, it's a new day, eh?" Kathy says. "If you have a laptop, I'll get the internet password for you. I know you can't sit up, but you could watch a show."

"That would be nice."

"Back when I started nursing, oh goodness, almost forty years ago now, it was a big deal to have televisions and phone lines in the rooms. Now, everyone needs the internet to keep them going. We still have some of those original bedside televisions to rent if you are interested."

"No, thanks. I'll be okay without TV."

"Figures. A hundred channels, and there's not much on anyway, is there?"

"Not really."

"*Brady Bunch. Mary Tyler Moore. Bonanza,*" Kathy says wistfully as she attaches a new IV bag to the pole. "Those were the golden years of television."

Kathy looks close to collecting her pension and, going by the generous volume of her bouffant, I guess that she came to her prime in the late sixties, dancing her way through nursing school with engineering students. Her hair, dyed a shade too dark, seems like a tribute to life before nightshifts and peewee soccer. Maybe she still taps her thumbs to the Bee Gees in her minivan as she drives to yet another twelve-hour shift.

"How was your night?" she asks. "Did you sleep?"

"A bit, here and there, thanks."

"You'll maybe get a nap this morning, something to help pass the time."

I groan on the inside. Is it as bad as all that? Sleeping to help pass the time is what old people do when they're waiting for Jesus to claim them: nap, watch a little *Jeopardy*, pick away at unappetizing food, and claim that time flies faster the older you get. Counting on a nap to move the day along feels so wasteful.

"The breakfast tray will be here shortly." Kathy eases a fresh pillow under my head. "If you need me, call."

"I'll be fine. I have Josh and he's fantastic."

"Lucky girl," she says, bustling out, hair bouncing.

Josh stretches out of his tightly coiled position. He swings his legs off the side of the chair-bed and rubs his eyes with his palms. He looks alarmingly disheartened.

"I know," I whisper. "It hits you all over again when you wake up."

He smiles wryly, then pads off to the washroom in bare feet. I can hear him yawning in the shower, but when he returns, ten minutes later, he looks energized.

"So, Amy," he says, standing at the end of my bed with his arms crossed over his damp white tee shirt, "we need names."

"I can't," I protest, waving a hand. "It takes too much effort."

"If the baby comes right away, we need a name."

I sigh. Naming the baby at this stage feels like giving a title to all the unhappiness we'll feel in the future. Whatever name we choose will forever be associated with our grief. Any child we meet with that name will remind us. But he's right. Picking names is something we can do to prepare.

"We've already talked about Andrew Lawrence to honour our deceased grandpas," I say. "How about Madeline if it's a girl?"

"Ma-de-line." Josh tries the name, perhaps listening for its natural flow. I think it rebounds beautifully, like a ball on a hardwood floor: "Ma," the initial strike; "da," the up-bounce; "line," the final resting place.

"I like it," he says. "But Madeline-what?"

"We'll keep thinking," I say, anxious to change the subject.

"Shall we talk about our plan if the baby doesn't make it?"

"I'm trying not to think about it," I say.

Josh sighs. "I was thinking of a burial."

"Maybe at home?"

"What? In Manitoba?" he asks.

"Yes. Years ago my great-grandmother lost four babies, one right after the other. They are buried beside her and Gramps in the old cemetery. I think the cemetery is filled now—they started a new plot on the other side of the road—but there might be room for another small grave beside Granny's babies."

The thought of those small headstones with a handful of days engraved on them is bleak but also a little soothing. Granny's large headstone casts a shadow over all the little ones.

"If that's what you want…okay," Josh says, "but then we'd both have to fly back to Manitoba for a burial. It would be more practical to have the grave here so we could visit more easily."

"True." I pull the bed sheet up to my mouth and envision cemetery visits. Perhaps we'd go every spring, hand in hand. We'd place a bundle of tulips beside a headstone with a concrete lamb on the top and, maybe, after a few years, our tears would flow less. It would be peaceful. The only sounds would be the rustle of tree branches over the markers of a thousand lives, old and young.

"It feels morbid to talk about burials," I say, trying to shake off the melancholy that has settled on us. This is only day two in hospital. Who knows what will happen?

• • •

A PAIN BEGINS AND THERE'S NOTHING SATISFYING ABOUT ITS agony. It's not like the first ten seconds of running or the gentle pressure of a good massage. It's a breathtaking twist in the middle of my stomach. I worry it's a contraction, even though I don't want to entertain the idea. Contractions mean labour, and labour at twenty-three weeks in the wrong hospital means disaster.

Josh reaches for the call button on my pillow, but I pull at his hand. "No. No. I'm fine," I say. "It's going away."

But a minute later, another pain comes, and then another. Official acknowledgement seems unavoidable, so Josh calls Nurse Kathy to my side.

She wraps a belt under me, then snaps it shut with a thick disc positioned over my belly button. The sound of the baby's heartbeat fills the room and Kathy nods in satisfaction.

"Baby is fine," she says. "Now I'm going to attach something to monitor contractions."

She snaps on a second belt as she did the first and watches the screen. "Any pain, Amy?" she asks.

"Not at the moment."

"Tell me when you feel something."

"I will," I say, but nothing comes. No twitching. No cramping.

Kathy waits, two minutes, then five, watching the screen, standing on one foot, then the other.

"You might feel pains that aren't contractions," she says. "Any pain could be within the realm of normal, considering the odd position you're lying in. Call me if it happens again and we'll try to track it."

She unsnaps the belt, then leaves with my medical chart under her arm. Josh pulls a chair close to my bed and wipes tears from my eyes with a balled-up Kleenex. He whispers something encouraging about how normal this all could be, but I'm not in the mood for placating.

"Bulging membranes aren't normal," I snap.

"I know," he soothes, "but it's going to take more than a few pains to produce the baby."

"Really? I nearly had the baby in a toilet yesterday."

He sighs and I feel guilty for being snippy. We need to support each other, but being told not to worry, not to be scared, just makes me more frantic. I need to prepare for the worst, not pretend that everything is going amazingly well.

I close my stinging eyes. A few pains aren't much, it's true, but now I want to reassess every decision we've made. If I am going into labour, how will I calmly push out a baby knowing we aren't going to resuscitate? A tiny baby, wrapped in a towel, growing ever more cold and still, a hand flexing, a tongue protruding—it will die like that. On my chest. Slipping from this world back to the one it came from.

I'm frightened, but I'm also angry. Perhaps it's my mothering instinct, or perhaps I am rallying enough strength to fight fate, because something inside of me clicks, and I know that no matter when the baby comes, we have to resuscitate. Today, tomorrow, whenever—we have to try to save the baby. I've lost patience with diagnoses and odds and percentages. If the baby dies, then at least we tried. If he or she lives and has disabilities, then we will cope. Besides, disabilities aren't the worst thing in the world. They are just disabilities. No better. No worse. We'll deal with them if we have to. I can't lie back anymore and let nature take its course. Nature is a shifty trickster anyway. It gets far too much applause for its dubious course that everything is supposed to take.

"Josh," I say, my eyes still closed, "I want to transfer."

"What? Now?"

"Yes, now. I want to transfer to the Grace Hospital now. I'm fed up with waiting. We have to be ready to resuscitate whenever the baby comes."

Josh pulls the chair closer, scraping the floor irritatingly. "You can't move if you are in labour, Amy."

"I'm not in labour. Isn't that what everyone keeps saying? Pains are normal, so let's go. I can't lie here knowing they can't resuscitate in this hospital. I can't."

I'm crying now, rather hysterically.

"Amy, don't get emotional!" Josh rubs my legs in long strokes, as if he can change my mind by soothing my body. "We made our decision based on the information given to us. We can't go changing course in the middle of things. What's this all about?"

"I can't push the baby out knowing that we're going to let it die," I sob. "It would be too sad. I can't."

"Okay, okay. Don't upset yourself." Josh leans over, kissing my forehead, smoothing down my ratty hair. I'm surprised to feel his hands shaking. I didn't think he was as susceptible to the effects of adrenaline as I am.

Another pain begins. Starting below my belly button, the pain spreads, fast enough for me to feel it unfurl, slow enough to stand the passing of time on its head.

Josh pushes the call button and Kathy comes quickly, nodding sagely at my wincing face. She clicks the monitor around my belly and, out of the corner of my eye, I can see a line on the monitor tracing a mountain like an Etch-a-Sketch drawing from my childhood toy box. The line jaggedly ascends, then avalanches as the pain ends.

"That was a contraction," Kathy says.

"I want to transfer to the Grace," I whisper.

"You have to wait until these contractions level off. They're not very regular, so there's a good chance they will stop altogether. I think you should wait until tomorrow morning at least."

I sniff back tears. I want to move today, not tomorrow.

"I know this is scary, Amy, but you don't want to have your baby on the side of the road, do you?"

"No."

"Okay then. I'll call the Grace Hospital to begin the arrangements, but you're not going today. No doctor will agree to a transfer in the middle of labour. Page me again if the pains become regular, even ten minutes apart."

Kathy leaves again, and Josh takes my hand.

"Why is this happening?" I sob.

"I'm frightened too, Babe," he says, "but your contractions aren't regular, so I'm sure they're going to stop."

"You don't know!"

"What else have we got, Amy? We have to think positively."

I cover my face with my one hand that isn't wired to the IV pole and wish I was somewhere else completely. Anywhere I don't have to lie still and wait for the next pain to stab through me. Somewhere the baby's life isn't in danger.

"Amy—do you want your mom to come?" Josh asks softly.

"Mom?" I sniff. "Why?"

"She's offered, and I think you need her."

"But it'll be so boring for her. Just bedside duty, running hot water bottles back and forth."

"She knows it's no holiday. So why not have her come?"

I picture the next few days. If I have the baby right away, I'm not sure I'll want Mom. I'll probably want to crawl into a corner and cry. But if I don't deliver right away and am flat on my back for ages, I might need someone to keep me sane.

"She won't annoy you?" I ask. "Mother-in-law and all that?"

"No. Of course not. I want you to be as relaxed as possible, and I think you need your mom. She'll help you to stay calm, not to panic."

"Oh, please." I roll my eyes. "I'm not panicking. Don't bug me."

"You're doing so well," Josh placates, "but I'm going to call her now and have her book a flight. Just rest a little."

Josh pecks my forehead, then disappears to the hall. And I glare up at the crooked, water-stained ceiling tiles for the thousandth time today. The room is quiet, but it's not peaceful. It's ominous. Everything is waiting. I breathe wafts of disinfecting hydrogen per-oxide, feel blood seep from me, and wish the madness was all over.

Chapter 8

DOUBTS PLAGUE ME. I FELT SO CONFIDENT WHEN I DEMANDED to be moved to the Grace but now, a day later, as I wait for the ambulance, I wonder if it's the best decision. Maybe some lives aren't meant to be saved. If we fight to keep our baby alive because we want a child and then it has a wretched life, isn't that selfishness? But if we let the baby drift off to sleep so we won't have to deal with disabilities, isn't that selfishness? Saving a life interferes as much as letting it go, and perhaps keeping a half-built baby alive for our pleasure is the very height of arrogant meddling.

And what is viability? That is a question that haunts me. Is viability a body kept alive by machines or is it a body capable of independent breath and thought? I don't know the answer, and medical advice is so speculative.

We're parents, not experts, yet we will decide how the odds will be played. Will we resuscitate only to be disappointed in the end, or will we let nature, in all its wretchedness, take its course? However bleak the predictions, at least if we resuscitate we won't have to wonder if the baby could have been saved. We will know. We will have tried. But still, I wish that I could ask the grown-up version of my unborn child what he or she wants. We're making decisions for that person too, the person that will live beyond us, who might be alone someday, without us. What does that person want?

So I lie fidgeting. As I wait for the paramedics to come, I pester Josh with questions: "Have you got my things packed? Our food out of the family fridge? Do you know how to get from here to the Grace Hospital?" I'm like a kid waiting to go on vacation, dressed and ready too early, driving everyone else in the house crazy.

The lunch cart has long since rattled back down the hall to the service elevators when three men in First Response uniforms traipse in, rolling a gurney between them. With crewcuts and slow drawls, they seem indistinguishable to me, though that could be because of my limited view.

"So...yep...we gotta get her on this stretcher," one of them says.

Josh eyes them carefully. "She's not allowed out of bed, you know," he says. "She should be lifted gently."

Nurse Janice sails into the room, barking orders: "Amy needs to be lifted onto the gurney as smoothly as you can. Do not jostle her. Be careful."

The paramedics all nod circumspectly, then position themselves on the three corners of my sheet with Josh at the fourth. One of them calls, "3! 2! 1! Up!" and suddenly I'm airborne, then down on the stretcher with a thud.

"Careful!" Janice snaps, grabbing my leg protectively.

"I'm fine, Janice," I mutter.

The paramedics set off toward the elevator with great speed, if not great finesse. Perhaps, if I had just suffered a car accident and a major artery was swiftly emancipating torrents of blood, I would have appreciated them dashing down the hall but, since I'm worried that a hearty sneeze may produce my baby, our bumpy journey concerns me.

Janice calls to the paramedics—"Lift her over the door frames, please!"—but she's largely ignored, so she runs ahead, throwing herself in front of obvious obstacles like corners, other stretchers, and a woman moaning on the bench outside Triage.

Down the hall, in an elevator, across the rotunda—as I'm pushed toward the hospital exit, I feel like I'm watching a movie trailer. One scene fades into another as people rush, caught up in their own dramas. A nurse calms an elderly woman who babbles incoherently, shaking a pill bottle in the air. A withered man slouches over in a wheelchair, waiting for something or someone to change his life while an oxygen line blisters his nose raw. People scurry. People scowl. No one seems to be enjoying their day at the hospital.

"Where are you parked?" Janice asks the paramedics.

"In the parking lot," says the one at the front as he steers my stretcher through the crowd.

"Why not under the covered Emergency entrance?"

"We save that for emergencies."

"But Amy is wearing a thin nightgown, and it's snowing!"

"We'll go quickly!" he says.

With that, I'm pushed out a double door, into the dismal March afternoon. Dusty clouds of gravel and ice pellets billow over asphalt. Low, ashen clouds mask an anaemic sky. My face stings from the cold as the paramedics dash the fifty feet to the waiting ambulance. I'm slid in head first and the doors are slammed. The last thing I see is Josh waving a faint goodbye with a grimacing smile.

• • •

"SO! THE HYPERTENSION GOTCHA, EH?"

The cheerful paramedic tries to defuse the tension that emanates from Janice's commanding presence as the two sit together on a narrow bench.

"Did you even read the chart?" Janice snaps. "She has bulging membranes, not hypertension, though she's likely to be tense by the end of this ride!"

"Okay. Sure. Bulging membranes…yep. Not good."

Undaunted, the paramedic presses on with lighter fare, safer topics such as the weather, the traffic, and the ubiquitous potholes of Canadian roads in spring. Janice ignores most of his chatter, but I find it diverting, almost calming. It's nice to have a normal conversation for twenty minutes, not one that's laced with dread and worry.

When we arrive at the Grace Hospital, Janice squeezes my hand. "It's been a pleasure to help you, Amy," she says.

"You've been so kind," I say, memorizing her face, as I'll probably never see her again.

She straightens up abruptly as the ambulance jolts to a stop. "I'll go up to the ward to make sure everything gets sorted," she says, looking pointedly at the paramedics, as if they are incapable of carrying charts to the correct counter.

I'm pulled out of the ambulance into a massive garage that echoes with CB radios and slamming doors. The paramedics shove my stretcher across the concrete floor while the narrow wheels squeak and turn all directions.

We pass two men being unloaded out of another ambulance. They look rough, homeless even. One holds a blood-soaked cloth to his head while the other rambles with jerky gesticulations, "No, I don't know what his real name is, see? He don't have a health card either. I'm his friend. But I don't know nothing, see?"

I'm pushed into the hospital through two glass doors which, oddly enough, sweep open into the psychiatric emergency ward. Perhaps the intricacies of efficient hospital design baffled the hospital's architect, but it seems unlikely that cutting a swath through Psych ER is the most peaceful way to usher an ailing patient into the Grace Hospital.

At the triage desk, a wild-looking man with matted hair screams at an unimpressed nurse. His saliva-spittled diatribe focuses on the tragedy of his hospitalization, the pointlessness of the endeavour, and the unkindness of all persons involved. The triage nurse holds her head in one hand and the phone in the other.

"Could you send someone down to help us with a situation?" she says into the receiver in a flat, tired voice.

"You're abusing me!" the man shrieks as we roll past.

The cheerful paramedic chirps back, "I'm abusing you? Wow! Bum luck you got, pal."

Janice pretends not to have seen or heard the interaction, and I suppose that despite preterm births, pregnancy losses, and full-term disasters, there are more challenging wards to work in than Labour and Delivery.

After a few turns and a long elevator ride with a cleaning lady and her wheeled mop pail, we end our journey in a Labour and Delivery room. I am returned to the Trendelenburg position and, after that, it's all old hat. My back seizes up and I can barely swallow. All the familiar faces disappear and the new ones just have questions.

• • •

AN OFFICIOUS, FRIZZY-HAIRED YOUNG MAN STRIDES INTO MY room without knocking or calling out the customary "Hello." I dislike him immediately.

"My name is Steven," he announces, as if Steven is the only name worth having. "I'm a second-year resident and I have some questions." He stands stiffly, his eyes darting nervously around the room, looking everywhere—at Josh, the bed sheets, the IV pole—everywhere but me.

"First, why are you here?" he asks.

"Why am I here?" I echo. "Have you got my chart from the Central?"

"Oh, yes. It's right here." He pats his clipboard with a patronizing smile.

"So what's your question?"

"Do you know why you're here? Do you understand everything that happened at the Central? I need to ask for clarification purposes."

"No problem." I say, then start a high-speed ramble: "I entered hospital two days ago with bulging membranes. I was at twenty-three weeks plus one day which makes me twenty-three plus three days, as of today."

He puts out his palm like a police officer might while directing traffic. "Twenty-three plus one, add two days. Right! That's twenty-three plus three."

"Great." I smile back at him and start in again: "I had an ultrasound at the Central which showed membranes bulging five to six centimetres beyond the cervix, ruling out a cervical cerclage. I was put in Trendelenburg position and have remained so since. We received counselling on premature birth outcomes and decided to resuscitate regardless of gestational age, which is why we transferred here."

I arch my eyebrows at him, waiting for him to catch up, but he is browsing through the many pages of my chart with a confused look on his face.

"And you're at twenty-three plus three?" he asks.

"Correct."

"Right. That's what your ultrasound report says as well."

"Oh, excellent."

"Any drug use, Amy?

"No."

"History of miscarried or terminated pregnancies?"

"No."

"A normal pregnancy before this?"

"Sure."

He slides his thick glasses up his nose with a strident middle finger and scans the chart for more information to clarify. "And your name is Amy Boyes?"

"It is." I sigh.

"That's all for now, but if I have any more questions, I'll be sure to come back."

As he leaves, he passes my chart to a petite, black nurse. When she introduces herself as Eileen, the soft sounds of the Jamaican shoreline come through in her accent.

"I see Steve has asked you every question in the world, so we're probably good there," she jokes.

"Unless you want me to confirm my gender?"

Eileen slaps her thigh, laughing. "Ah! That's a good one. I know those questionnaires are the limit, but they eliminate confusion, even if their side effect includes hypertension."

She points to Josh—"Husband?"—so he quickly stands and introduces himself.

"How does he put up with you?" she teases.

"No idea," I fire back.

"Well, Amy, hopefully you're going to lie here for a long time before your baby comes but, on the chance you don't, we're going to do a steroid shot for baby's lungs development and then more counselling. I know you talked to Dr. Shumar at the Central, but Dr. Hudson will see you too. Seth is a senior fellow, almost a full-fledged neonatologist. We're also going to get you on a magnesium drip with a saline solution."

"Why magnesium?

"Some studies show it reduces uterine activity, holds off preterm birth."

"When do I get the steroid shot?"

"Right now," she says, holding up a needle. "And it's fanny-first, so roll over."

I snicker, then slowly turn onto my right side, exposing my posterior through the opening of the rather inadequate nightgown.

"Three...two..." Eileen stabs in the needle and I gasp in pain.

"Yep! That one burns for some reason," she chuckles. "I try not to warn patients too much. Makes you nervous, and how would that help?"

Eileen wheels an IV pole with a saline bag swinging on it to my left side and fishes out another needle from her cart. "Don't worry, I'll be careful with this one."

I stretch out my left arm and look out the window to distract myself from the blood work. My view is limited to grey clouds, a disadvantage of my reclined position and of being on the hospital's eighth floor in an otherwise residential neighbourhood.

"I have to tell you, Amy, this magnesium is going to sting in your veins," Eileen warns. "I got it up to room temperature so it won't be too bad, but if it comes straight out of the fridge, oh boy, you'll be crying."

Eileen starts the IV pump, and I feel a rush of cold pain. I picture ice spreading through my arm like an arctic volcano filling gorges and valleys. If this bag is at room temperature, then straight out of the fridge must be breathtaking.

"Have you always worked in Labour and Delivery, Eileen?" I ask, trying to distract myself from the pain that speeds down my arm and into my shoulder.

"Yes and no. I started in Maternity in England where I studied after emigrating from Jamaica, but when my husband got a job in Ottawa I worked in Emergency."

"This ward must be like Emergency sometimes, no?"

"Depending on the day, sure. It's not too bad at the moment. We've got twins who can't make up their minds whether to stay or come, a woman breathing in sync with Enya, and a few others in various stages."

I like Eileen. She is plain-speaking and funny and, like Janice at the Central, doesn't bother with too much knee-patting.

"Do you get many premature babies?" Josh asks.

"Oh, sure. All the time."

"As early as twenty-three weeks though?"

"Some. We get twins and triplets more and, though they're not always extremely premature, they can be high-risk in other ways."

Eileen unravels the same thick belt with a disc that was used at the Central and, after fastening it around my stomach, plugs it into a monitor, then listens. There's only silence, so Eileen slides the wand a little to the right, a little to the left, but still there's only silence. Finally, she locates the baby's heartbeat in the bottom of my stomach. Nodding in satisfaction, she unclips the apparatus.

"My goodness, that baby is low," she says.

"What does that mean?" I ask.

"The baby is small, for one thing. There hasn't been time for it to grow very big. The other thing, of course, is what we already know— your cervix is completely dilated and the membranes are emerging from your body. The baby is very nearly born, so it sits low, ready to appear."

I'm silent, almost sorry I asked the question.

Eileen enquires about our families—are they close? Are they upset by this development? She seems satisfied with our answers, especially when I say that my mother arrives this afternoon. Perhaps Eileen's job is made easier when a patient is accompanied by an older woman, someone who has given birth herself and isn't easily put off. If nothing else, Mom can make tea and straighten my bed covers, freeing Eileen to monitor patients who are actually in labour.

Eileen asks what brought us to Ottawa, and we recount our tale of jumping at job opportunities—Josh leaving the prairies for work in the House of Commons; me starting the teaching studio—a tale somewhat similar to her own, if two Atlantic crossings are disregard-ed. Her history is a classic first-generation immigrant story (work hard, big moves); ours, more like a tale of moderately achieving, sixth-generation Canadians. In comparison to Eileen's, our pasts aren't very dramatic; our actions, not so desperate.

"Do you ever visit Jamaica?" Josh asks.

"My husband goes every year for a couple of months, but I only go for a week or two," Eileen answers. "Can't stand the sitting around in the heat! Two days and I'm bored."

"Tell me about it," I mutter.

"Oh, Sugar!" Eileen laughs. You're gonna get a lot more bored than this. I'll make it my mission to keep you here till this baby grows some lungs, and in the meantime you're gonna lose your mind! Wait for it."

She leaves the room in the easy saunter of someone raised in the tropics and I stare up at the ceiling, hoping for something interesting to look at. I'm rewarded with a koala—not an actual picture of a cuddly, dark-eyed koala, but rather a smudge of water damage in the shape of a koala, recognizable only if squinted at. And I do squint at it—repeatedly, in fact—until my blood-rushed head hurts worse than ever.

• • •

MY CELLPHONE BEEPS WITH A MESSAGE FROM MOM: "AT GATE. Can hardly wait to get there."

I picture Mom, waiting for her early morning flight, exhausted from a restless night at the airport hotel in Winnipeg. She can't sleep in a strange bed, never could. When I was a kid, she always spent the first night of vacations listening to Dad snore and me sleep talk, wondering why she even bothered.

She's a trouper to come at a moment's notice. Goodness knows, the ticket couldn't have been cheap. And poor Dad. He's probably already lonely, driving away from the airport across the flat, prairie farm land, feeling badly about all this drama in Ottawa.

My parents are making quite an effort for me, so I resolve to be nicer to them. I'm not a hideous child, at least I don't think so, but I'm not amazingly supportive either. I have a bad habit, honestly inherited from my Northern Irish ancestors, of saying precisely what I think. My parents resent the habit, despite being its genetic source, never once appreciating me sorting out their nonsense, their foibles, their nervous opinions. A typical conversation with my parents involves dire warnings from them—"Forget RRSPs, get your money in gold, Amy," or "Diclectin is dangerous; try a bit of ginger for your morning sickness instead"—and dismissive rebuttals from me. But it does seem that they are growing increasingly wary as they age, less trusting, more nervous. They believe all governments lie and newspapers fictionalize, all food not produced on one's own farm is cancer-causing, and all cities are crime-ridden dens of iniquity. Their theories are just true enough to be difficult to argue against, and the severity of their opinions seem to grow in direct proportion to the improving speed of their rural internet.

It's an age-old scenario though: child thinks parents senile; parents think child reckless. Both, of course, know they're right. But even in the midst of our complex relationship, my parents and I have an inescapable bond. Like a scene from a *National Geographic* documentary where the mother elephant barrels through the bamboo to rescue her distressed baby, my mother purchased an expensive, last-minute ticket to fly over the Boreal Shield just to get to me. Unlike the mother elephant, she can't save me from my distress, but she'll at least try to make it better.

I hear the hospital room door open.

"I'm back, Babe!" Josh calls out. He holds a paper bag and a cup of tea from the Second Cup in the lobby. He hands me a warm butter croissant and I very nearly inhale the flakey, buttery chunks. "Sorry, crumbs in the sheets will probably drive you mad."

"Thank you, my darling," I murmur, only now realizing how hungry I am.

Josh always used to bring me food in bed. When we were first married, he'd get up early on the weekend and then sneak back to bed with a tray of fresh bread the way I like it, lightly toasted and buttered, and a mug of coffee. I'd sit up, leaning against the headboard, pretending I couldn't see anything without my contact lenses, and then would act shocked to see the tray under my nose. Josh would snuggle in beside me, pleased as a school boy on trphy day to see me happy.

"Josh, stop bumping, you scoundrel!" I'd joke as he'd try to kiss me around my coffee mug. "It's indecent to ply me with breakfast, then take advantage of my gratitude!"

This past winter, Josh brought me dishes of breakfast food designed to satisfy the fickleness of my nauseous stomach—a few crackers, a slice or two of cheese, a couple of grapes, all laid out in perfect symmetry on a dessert plate, but there was never a drop of gag-inducing coffee in sight. He would kiss my cheek, then slip off to work, leaving me to sleep. And now, in the middle of a Labour and Delivery ward, he feeds me again, but there is no jostling horseplay, no cheerful kissing, no jokes or cuddles. It's all so deadly serious.

Chapter 9

DR. HUDSON HAS FRECKLES SPRINKLED ACROSS A BABY-FACE, which give him boy-like look, though he must be nearly forty. Other than the freckles, his skin is pale from a winter inside the hospital, though most of us white Canadians are pasty by March, indoor work or not.

He shakes Josh's hand and awkwardly waves at me in lieu of what might have been an even more awkward handshake. I raise my eyebrows with what I hope is taken as a wry appraisal of the situation, not a spasm in my upper face. Lying in Trendelenburg—head down, feet in the air—throws a curveball into social conventions.

Dr. Hudson finds a stool and wheels it to the end of my bed. I can see him if I roll my eyes to their extreme southerly position, but the effort causes a sharp pain in my head, so I give up and stare at the koala on the ceiling instead.

"I know you talked with Dr. Shumar at the Central," the doctor begins, "so a lot of what I'm going to say will be familiar. I've brought some literature which shows the average outcomes for the extremely premature births in Ottawa for the last ten years."

I let myself tune out. I don't want to hear it all again, the horrid numbers, the percentages, the averages, the likelihoods. What are we? Bookies? How can we make decisions based on numbers from a big white binder? It is all well and good to say that X number of cases end well and X number end poorly, but what about our case? How will it end? No one knows, so I see no reason to listen to the grim discussion all over again. We've made our decision and more talking won't change our minds.

Dr. Hudson goes on and on in a gentle voice, often stopping to nod and purse his lips as if to affirm his words. Josh listens and then, in his infuriating habit, repeats everything just to be sure he understands. I want to shush them both: the doctor for saying horrible things about death and disabilities, and Josh for repeating it as if once wasn't enough. As my annoyance with the men increases, so does the pain in my back. The thin labour room mattress isn't intended for a long-term stay and the pain makes me claustrophobic.

I need a cry too—a drippy, ugly-faced cry, the kind they never show in movies because they are too hideous for the screen—but I decide to save it for later when I'll be alone. I don't want the doctor sending up the psychologist because I lost it in front of him. "A nice chat" would seriously finish me.

Just as I wonder if the conversation will ever end, Josh sums up our decision: we will resuscitate; if the heart is not beating, we will not do compressions and the baby will be returned to our room for comfort care. Otherwise, every attempt should be made to save the life.

Dr. Hudson nods cheerfully, as if he's relieved. I wonder if he was hoping we'd choose resuscitation despite his bleak explanation of the literature. He doesn't seem to wish we'd give up so an incubator can be saved for a baby with a better chance of survival. In fact, he seems pleased with our faith in the system, our confidence in his and his colleagues' ability to save our child's life.

"Hopefully, we'll never need to act on these decisions," he says. "Maybe the baby won't come for weeks."

"Wouldn't that be nice?" I say, wondering how I'll survive. Time moves so slowly that just watching the clock's long hand makes one rotation feels like a full day's work. I won't be able to cope with weeks, let alone months, of bed rest. But what other option do I have?

The doctor leaves, and for a moment Josh and I silently watch each other, again musing about the horrible facts of a counselling session. We feel the responsibility of our decisions. We're toying with another life, making decisions for a third person who can't voice an opinion but will have to live with the consequences.

"What a day," Josh eventually says, leaning back into the easy chair, shutting his eyes.

"Agreed," I murmur, but I keep my eyes open. I'm scared of sleeping during the day; nights are so endless. I need to keep awake, so I try to read, but the IV line tugs painfully as I hold a book and my declined head hurts when I focus on words. I call my sister and grandmother, but there's no news from either of them, so the calls are short. I read the news on my phone, but the cell service is poor and the mobile pages jam. I give up and go back to watching the koala on the ceiling.

When I was a kid on the farm, hours and hours of my summers were spent weeding, mowing, or picking whatever crop was in season. There was nothing quite like fifty feet of green beans under a scorching sun with mosquitoes swarming to motivate an escapist imagination. I would dream up wild adventures—I was a pioneer kid, a slave dreaming an escape to Canada on the underground railway, an Olympian competing in an epic bean-picking event. My imaginings worked—I survived the boredom of farm work—so now, in the middle of a hospital, twenty-odd years later, I try calling upon my imagination to picture beautiful days with a baby who I hope will live to see them, but even that is difficult.

It seems I've lost patience with dreaming of unlikely things. It's wasteful. Besides, an Olympic bean-picking competition as a ten-year-old is one thing, but an epic three-month Olympic bed-resting competition at twenty-seven is another. I'm too depressed for positive thinking.

• • •

MOM SAILS INTO MY HOSPITAL ROOM IN HER LAVENDER WOOL coat, silver-flecked scarf flowing behind her. "Oh, Amy!" she gasps. "It's lovely to see you, but wow—you look rough!"

"I feel rough, actually. How was your flight?"

"Fine, fine. A bit of turbulence at the end, but nothing too bad."

Mom presses her soft, cool cheek comfortingly against mine. A tear rolls out of her eye, and I suppose I do look pitiful. I haven't combed my hair in three days and any makeup has long since worn off. I feel greasy and bloated. But I'm pleased to see my mother. My bravery and resolve are slipping as my hospitalization moves into its third day and, simply put, I want my mom. I want her to take control of the untidy room and cheer me up like she did when I was a child, always seeing the bright side of things, not allowing me to wallow in self-pity.

Mom is short and spunky. Her curly hair clenches into spirals in humidity, making her look a bit like Shirley Temple, all grown up. Her eyes are a pretty shade of green, but they're set behind glasses, placed under a demonstrative pair of eyebrows. Mom's changing moods can be monitored through close observation of said eyebrows. In a neutral position, one has nothing to fear. In a lowered, furrowed position, fast explaining is required. In a high, arched position, all is lost.

Hands on hips, eyebrows high, she looks at me squarely. "Your face is awfully swollen," she says.

"I expect it's the bed rest. Fluid retention and all that."

"I once got a steroid shot for asthma and my face ballooned. Have they given you steroids?"

"One for the baby's lungs, but I expect the puffiness is nothing."

"Have you asked them about it?"

"No, I'm fine."

Mom huffs in Josh's direction, "Okay, Husband—are you going to talk to the nurses about the puffiness if she won't?"

"Possibly," he says with mock serenity and a vague gesture. He rarely wanders into an argument between Mom and me.

"Can I get you anything?" she asks me.

"A refill on the hot water bottles would be nice," I puff. My back is aching, and no matter how hard I try I can't get a good gulp of air. Breathing has been difficult since I went on bed rest—it's like working against gravity—but it's getting worse as the days go by.

Mom lets the water run in the sink a solid two minutes before she fills the hot water bottles. They burn a little as she wedges them under my back with only my thin nightgown protecting me from the hot rubber, but they'll be cool again in ten minutes, so I don't mention it.

"I feel bad for all this fuss, Mom."

"Don't. I wanted to come."

"Have a seat, eh?"

Mom sits beside me and tells me all the news from home. She and Dad want to redo their kitchen, but new cupboards are a fortune. They may just do the backsplash and the countertops instead. She tries to draw me in—"What do you think of a brown rock pattern for the counters? Too dark?"—and says how concerned my sisters, Mavis and Maureen, are for me. She tells me about my nieces' and nephews' accomplishments in a proud but cautious voice, and her worries for the younger generation are mirrored in her concern for the older: Grandpa's eyes are very bad. One grandma has been diagnosed with dementia; the other has bad feet, an unsteady gait.

Mom peppers the conversation with stories she's already told me, some multiple times, a habit she finds unspeakably frustrating in others. I stare up at my water-stain koala and wonder if there is a magic tipping point in life—a place where all of your best experiences lie behind. Popular thought says that you never stop learning, but it doesn't seem that way. It seems that at some point, you stop re-evaluating. You live with whatever accomplishments you've achieved and let the rest go.

But even though I know my mother's opinions on every topic before she says them, I'm glad to listen to her. She is comforting, exactly what a mother should be.

When nurses come and go, Mom chats easily with them, asking all sorts of questions about their careers and families. Within an hour, they are all fast friends, firing off crazy patient stories across my bed. Mom keeps up her end with tales from her days as a medical receptionist and by the time the supper cart comes with some appalling offering I'm already in a better mood. Mom's presence has rallied me and I'm grateful for it. She makes sure Josh eats properly, goading him into cleaning up my supper tray, then visiting the cafeteria for a decent bite. She finds the family kitchen and boils water for tea, fixing Josh's exactly how he likes it. When she finally puts her feet up, she retrieves a pad of paper from her purse and begins a shopping list.

"We're going to assume that you will find every meal as objectionable as you did supper tonight," she says. "We need a plan to keep up your energy and fill you with fibre. Now, what appeals?"

"Deli ham with aged white cheddar on white bread."

Mom rolls her eyes. "Fibre! Fibre, I tell you! How else will you move your intestines along?"

"I'm not going to 'move my intestines', as you so delicately put it. It's what nearly produced the baby, and since the poor thing is hanging on with its fingernails, I'm not bothering again."

"Don't be silly. You have to, and if you don't you'll be in pain. That's why your stomach hurts."

"It doesn't hurt."

"It will soon."

She writes items in her perfect cursive handwriting that makes mine looks like the work of an arthritic ape in a hurry.

"I'll write down whole wheat tortilla wraps instead of bread, and you'll get a sliver of cheese if you promise to eat some dried prunes," she says.

"Oh, for crying out loud!"

"It's for your own good. Would you eat yogurt?"

"I suppose."

"I'll get you some with fibre pellets in it."

"Sounds amazing."

"Don't be smart. You'll need all the help you can get. Maybe Josh can go for these things in the morning."

"He probably needs out. He's been so good to me." I smile in the direction of my husband snoozing in the lounge chair.

"From the moment he first called, I could hear the concern in his voice," Mom says. "Can you imagine not being able to count on him in a time of crisis?"

"He's so caring. He doesn't think of himself as a kind person, but he is. His cousin says that when she was a kid, she was scared of Josh's farm dog, which I can hardly blame her for—they keep such nippy dogs, for some reason—so Josh used to meet her at the car door, take her by the hand and lead her around the yard so she wouldn't be frightened. There must have been a lot of kindness in a little boy who would do that."

Mom fusses some more about my swollen face and ragged breathing, then kisses me goodbye. Her ride, a kind neighbour of ours, has arrived to take her to our house for the night.

As she leaves, I feel a little panicked. I don't want her to go, not even for the night. After all the years Mom and I have lived apart, it's odd I have separation anxiety now, but maybe stress has brought it on.

"See you in the morning," I call after her, trying to push my childish instinct into a little corner of my mind, but the evening has lost its warm glow of storytelling and pleasant conversation. I start to worry about what tomorrow might bring.

• • •

SOMEONE IS IN MY ROOM. IT'S DARK, BUT I CAN TELL THE SHADowy figure attaching something to my IV pole isn't Bonnie, my night nurse. Bonnie carried my IV bags under her arm to warm them before attaching them to my pole. This strange nurse is in a hurry.

"Sorry!" she whispers. "I've come with a fresh bag of magnesium."

I mumble something about warming the bags, but I'm too tired to speak clearly, so the nurse pats my hand and leaves. I squint at the wall clock, but I can't make out the difference between the tall and short hands. Is it 4:15 or 3:20? I'm not sure.

Some loose bits of mucus start whistling in Josh's nose, so he stirs, smacking his lips and snoring again, softly at first, then more adamantly. I wish we were in bed at home, my back against his chest, his kisses on my neck. No more pain. No more staring at the ceiling. I'd be cozy, safe.

I drift back to sleep and dream I'm a kid, back on the farm. It's a wonderful late-summer afternoon with a hint of wheat dust in the air from the combines. I'm reading *Pygmalion* in my favourite tree behind the raspberry patch, wishing someone would recreate me, eradicating my stringy hair and juvenile awkwardness, making me pretty like Eliza.

Suddenly, a mosquito bites my arm. I swat it, but it keeps biting, harder and harder. I swat it again and again, but the pain gets worse. I cry out and a voice cuts through my dream.

"Amy! Wake up!" Josh is hovering over me, brushing my bangs off my forehead.

"A mosquito bit me," I cry.

"No, Love, it's March. A mosquito didn't bite you. Stop hitting yourself."

He yanks the little string to the light behind my bed, and for a moment we blink at each other in the brightness, then at my arm. It's nearly twice its normal size, tight and red, and excruciatingly painful.

Josh pushes the nurse's call button. "Bonnie, please!"

Within seconds, Bonnie is in the room, shaking her head. "Your IV line is unloading into your arm tissues, not your vein. That's why your arm is so swollen."

She moves quickly, gently detaching the IV from my arm. She touches the magnesium bag and gasps—"I'm so sorry! This bag is stone-cold. I forgot to remind my break nurse to warm it. Here, Josh, take the bag and warm it under your arm."

She unhooks the bag of fluid and Josh stuffs it under his pajama top.

"You're feeling both the cold magnesium and the pressure of the IV going interstitial," Bonnie explains. "Your arm will feel better, but it's going to take a while. I'm going to put a new needle in your other arm. Hold your left arm still. That's it! Three…two…one!"

Bonnie eases a needle into the inside of my left elbow. The prick hurts less than I expect it to. In fact, all needles hurt less than they did a day or two ago. Perhaps everything else is hurting more or perhaps I'm distracted by the bits of gravel that seem to have filled my lungs. For some reason, I don't tell Bonnie how difficult breathing has become. I just let her finish the IV, shut off the light and disappear.

"Are you cold, Amy?" Josh whispers in the darkness.

"A bit."

He pulls my black wool winter coat from the wardrobe and spreads it over my legs. The coat lies heavily over me, keeping the draft from the window at bay.

"Go back to sleep, Love," I say. "I'm sorry to have woken you."

With no further ado, Joes lies back on his pullout bed and is sleeping soundly within minutes, snoring hearty drags through his nose.

The cool cloth that Bonnie wrapped around my swollen arm slips onto my stomach, soaking my thin nightgown. I fling the cloth impatiently onto the bed rail and try to ignore the fire in my arm, but there's nothing else to think about. After closing my eyes for what feels like a long time, I squint at the clock and see that it's only 3:36, a mere sixteen minutes after I first woke. I wonder how it's possible for time to creep this slowly. I'm in so much pain. I want to claw at something. I want to scream. I want to get up and walk out of the hospital.

But since panic doesn't help, I try to think of something cheerful, something distracting. I picture bringing the baby home, even though there's a good chance the baby won't survive. I imagine the baby running and jumping and playing like every other child, but those wretched numbers in the binders worry me. I think about teaching, but wonder if I'll want to teach kids if my baby dies or if we'll be able to find child care if the baby is disabled. I think of a summer vacation. If the baby survives, we certainly won't take one, but if the baby doesn't survive, a change of scenery might do us good. Maybe we'll go somewhere relaxing. A walking tour of rural England. The Balkans. Josh has expressed an interest in Croatia. Exploring old Dubrovnik. Why not? I think of our bank account balance. It isn't so good.

My friend Michael has agreed to teach my piano studio during my hospitalization. He's taking a year between university degrees, so he's available and cash-strapped. It's gracious of him to step into my shoes but expensive for me. I'll be paying him with money already spent on bills.

It's funny how I never used to worry about money. Even as a broke student, a lack of money was a secondary concern. All I worried about was keeping up with my work load. That was what interested me. Within the practice rooms of music school, I learned the thrill of achievement. It was the adrenaline I craved. Changing my life, one term at a time, was deeply satisfying.

But now I'm worried. Lying in hospital for unknown lengths of time feels wasteful, destructive even. All my drive has vanished. The forward momentum I've carefully honed over the last ten years is slowly disintegrating, depreciating in value. I feel desperate for change, but seemingly incapable of producing it.

Chapter 10

"SHE'S NOT GOING TO EAT ANY OF THIS," MOM MUTTERS AS SHE RAKES over the breakfast tray.

"Try me," I yawn.

"Oh, good morning. There's cold, grey porridge, a clump of scrambled eggs, and a piece of cardboard trimmed into the general shape of a slice of bread," she says cheerfully.

"Yeah, no. I don't want any of it."

"No matter. I stopped at Second Cup and got you a croissant with cheddar cheese. What do you think?"

"I think you are marvellous."

"You'll have to counter-balance all the white flour with a hearty prune intake."

Mom fishes my contact case out of the night-stand and helps me line up the flimsy bits of hydrogel lenses with my eyes. The lenses are slippery and one falls off my finger as I hold it above my face. She gently picks the lens off the pillow and we begin again.

The contact lenses clarify what I already saw through blurred vision: Josh is still asleep on the fold-out chair; it's a grey, dismal day; and my arm is still swollen. I wave it at Mom like a kid with a boo-boo.

"Looks awful. What happened?" she asks.

"The IV line popped out of my vein, unloaded into my arm. Hurts like the dickens."

"I bet. Finish that croissant and I'll fix your hair."

I touch the back of my head. "Rat's nest" seems an apt description.

"Don't worry about it," I mumble, but Mom gives me a dark eye.

"You needn't go to pieces because you're on bed rest; besides, here you are, twenty-three weeks plus four days and you haven't gone into labour. That's lots to be thankful for."

"I know," I say, still glum.

"Now, Michael is coming to talk about your teaching schedule this morning, so we need to fix you up. Hair, mascara, the lot. You'll feel better and won't scare Michael."

Michael and I first met as undergrad piano majors. I had a nervous stomach; Michael, a permanent twitch. We lived in constant fear of failure and poverty. Undoubtedly, we would have suffered a lifetime of that if we had pursued careers as performers, but we wisely chose other specializations in our graduate degrees: I, piano pedagogy; Michael, musicology. Our shared anxiety forged a strong bond though. We're still friends years later, and I appreciate him teaching my studio while I'm in hospital.

I don't feel like fixing up and even protest against it, but thankfully Mom proceeds, because when Michael tiptoes into the room, clutching a bundle of white daisies by their stems, thrusting them forward as if to ward off danger, he stares with wide-eyed amazement. Hair combed or not, I seem to alarm him.

"Michael." I motion to the flowers. "You shouldn't have!"

"How are you? How are you?"

He rushes over, but doesn't seem to know if he should pat my shoulder, kiss my cheek or hold my hand. He doesn't manage any of the gestures well, but I understand. He's trying to comfort me, but he's never had a pregnant friend in crisis before and the chill of the hospital room alarms him.

I try to put Michael at ease but, as I repeat my tale of woe, it seems unbelievable even to me that I'm in danger of giving birth sixteen and a half weeks early. The story upsets me, and Michael shakes his head and pats my hand as I talk. I frequently stop to gulp air because the feeling of gravel in my lungs is getting worse.

Mom eyes me suspiciously as she hands me the teaching schedule she brought from home that morning. "Slow down, Amy," she says. "Take your time."

"Do Ella and Olivia's ear training and theory together," I puff. "They're sisters so they come at the same time and are at the same level. Besides, who wants to explain augmented intervals twice in one day? Be careful—Jocelyn's understanding of rhythm is shaky. It won't be enough just to correct errors. Help her subdivide or you'll get to hear the same mistakes next week. Don't let Lucy talk her whole lesson or you'll get nothing done. She has a new sight-reading book. It's on my desk—you'll see it—and her mother owes $10 for it. Please remind her every lesson until you see the $10. Sorry, it's a pain, but it's the job. James is a bit of a know-it-all so take no guff; I never do. He's super-talented, thank goodness, or he'd be unspeakably annoying."

I go on and on, breathing harder and faster as I describe the management of forty-five students. I explain parents and personalities, lesson plans and expectations. Michael scribbles notes in the margins of the schedule, but I know I'm overloading him with details. I can barely keep track and I've seen these kids once a week for years. Nevertheless, he just has to keep everyone motivated through year-end recitals, competitions, and exams. His teaching experience is limited, but he's patient. He'll be fine.

After an hour, he leaves, awkwardly patting, kissing, hugging me again. It's only midday, but I'm completely exhausted.

"You talked too much," Mom says. "You're beat."

"I can't get my breath," I say, shifting slightly onto my left side, trying to ease my back pain. Suddenly, I can't breathe at all. It's as if massive paws grip my chest, squeezing the air out of me. I roll onto my back and gasp at the ceiling.

"Amy! Are you okay?" Josh calls from the easy chair.

"I can't breathe. On my side...nothing."

Mom and Josh stumble over each other to hit the nurse's call button. When Nurse Eileen appears, they speak evenly but quickly—"Can't breathe on her side. Tires easily."

Eileen clips an oxygen saturation sensor onto my finger and plugs the other end of the cord into a monitor. She watches my vitals on a screen with her hands on her hips and shakes her head.

"This machine can't be working," she says, staring at the blinking number. "I'm going to grab a different machine."

Eileen retrieves a new oxygen saturation monitor and two residents from the hallway. She deftly sets up the new machine—lines draped over the bed rail, into the machine, out it again, and into the wall—and when it beeps to life, they all gasp.

"Eighty?" whispers one of the residents.

"We need Dr. Ahmed," Eileen says, then dashes from the room. One resident shifts the sensor from one of my fingers to the next, trying to get a better number, though no particular finger changes the expression on her face.

A doctor, presumably Ahmed, strides into the room, snapping, "Get her on oxygen now and lift her into a sitting position."

But we all freeze—Mom, Josh, Eileen, the nurses. His advice is opposite to what we've been told.

"No! Absolutely not," I argue. "I have bulging membranes so I have to be kept flat!"

Eileen fastens an oxygen mask over my face, effectively ending my protests, but she doesn't lift my bed. Like Mom and Josh, she stares the doctor down, wondering if his orders should be followed or fought. He senses the opposition.

"Look!" he says, a vein bulging on his forehead. "If she's not breathing, the baby's not breathing. We don't even know that bed rest is keeping the baby inside. She has very bad oxygen saturation, and we don't know why. We have to get her breathing, so turn up the oxygen and get her into a sitting position."

Eileen hits a lever and I feel my head rise. Mom holds my hand, but I wrench it away, ripping the oxygen mask off my face. Shaking with adrenaline, I level at the doctor, "I want a second opinion! I have been told to stay with my head down and now you are lifting me? No! Stop it!"

"Shhh. Shhh." Eileen pats my hand and lifts me an inch or two further.

"More," says the doctor when Eileen stops. She hits the lever again, but only for a second. "Amy, you have to understand," he says pleadingly. "Your oxygen levels are very low, and the baby receives all of its oxygen from you. If your oxygenation is not optimized then neither is the baby's. Please, put the mask back on."

Josh stands at the foot of my bed, eyes wide, arms crossed. Our eyes meet and communicate fear. I put the mask back on my face and breathe a few breaths.

"Eight-two," Eileen calls.

"That isn't fast enough," says the doctor. "Can you turn up the oxygen?"

"A bit." She turns the dial and a stronger breeze fills the mask.

"Why did this happen?" Mom asks quietly.

"Hard to say," the doctor says. "It's most likely a reaction to the steroid shot for the baby's lungs. It can cause maternal fluid retention. Of course, it doesn't help Amy is in Trendelenburg; that position makes it hard for the lungs to clear. We'll give her some Lasix to help drain the extra fluid from her body."

"Eight-three," Eileen says, giving the breeze in my mask yet another hike. The doctor nods approvingly and walks out, leaving Eileen to monitor me.

"I'm nervous, Eileen," I say, lifting my mask for a second.

"It's okay, Amy. Put the mask back on. Dr. Ahmed has zero bedside manner, but he's a good doctor. He doesn't give bad advice. I know this is a reversal from what you were originally told, but the situation has changed. Once we get your oxygen saturation back up, we can always lower you again."

By the time Eileen says "Eight-six," I'm losing steam. I've toppled off my surge of adrenaline and feel bad for snapping at the doctor who was only trying to help. I close my eyes and focus on breathing, in and out, against the flow. The oxygen in the mask reminds me of a prairie wind.

As a kid, I would bicycle north, into a wind that had already rolled over a continent of undulating nothingness before blowing right up our farm road, into my face. The wind would pelt dust into my eyes and tangle my fine hair, but I would pedal into it anyway, always in a big hurry to get to the end of the road so I could bike back to the yard with the wind pushing me home. I imagine I'm biking into that breeze now, defying nature—"Take that, wind! You don't slow me down!"—but somewhere along the ride, maybe halfway down the lane, I fall asleep. Mom holds my hand. Josh paces.

• • •

WHEN I WAKE, THE OXYGEN FLOW IN MY MASK HAS BEEN RE-duced from a prairie windstorm to a gentle breeze. Through heavy eyelids, I see Josh on the fold-out chair reading Dr. Hudson's litera-ture and Mom texting furiously like a teenager with a secret.

I lift my oxygen mask. "Can I have some water?" I whisper hoarsely.

Mom holds a cup of ice water beside my chin and points the straw toward my mouth. I suck back and feel the iciness slosh down to my stomach.

I think of suffering through flu bugs as a child. I would lie like this, on the couch, eating strawberry Jell-O, sipping from a colourful straw. This plain white straw makes me wish for the cheerful can-dy-striped straw from years ago.

I refasten the oxygen mask. "Who are you texting?" I ask Mom in a muffled voice.

"Your dad," she says. "He's concerned about this fluid business."

"Don't upset him," I mumble. "We're getting it sorted."

"Your catheter bag is almost full since they gave you the Lasix. It's mostly clear, straight fluid pouring out of you. You must have had a pile of water on board. No wonder you're thirsty; everything is draining."

I still feel sleepy—the stress of the afternoon exhausted me—but now that I'm lying more upright, I have a better view out the window. I watch as the fading afternoon sun spreads a golden sheen across the tops of buildings. Headlights on the Queensway streak across the dusky horizon and streetlights pop on across the city, one neigh-bourhood at a time.

After days of staring at the ceiling, I'm surprised to see my toes peeking out from under my blanket. Although scarlet polish flakes off my nails as it did before my hospitalization, my feet now look foreign to me, like a pan shot of an actor's feet in a movie. They don't seem like mine. I can't touch or scratch them without scrunching and stretching and I wouldn't dare do that. I'm at the mercy of others to cover my feet with socks or blankets. Although they are connected to me, I'm disconnected from them. My torso belongs to me—I can feel its bumps and curves—but I share it with the medical professionals. Strangers yet strangely intimate, they monitor, listen, prod, and scan. Nothing is off-limits to the instruments they carry: the slippery ultrasound wand, the pinching catheter line, the snug transducer belt, or even the frosty stethoscope. All is exposed. My arms are wired to an IV pole and even my poor, needle-pricked backside has had its moment in the sunshine. All that belongs to me is my face, but with the oxygen mask strapped on I've lost it too. I'm reduced to a pair of ears and eyes, listening and watching around elastic straps, tracking worried faces, ignoring the dawdling clock, tuning in and out of conversations as I please. I'm both trapped inside my body and divorced from it.

When the supper cart arrives, Eileen brings nasal oxygen prongs so I can eat and turns down the oxygen flow even further.

"Good girl, Amy," she says. "You're breathing much better and your face is certainly less swollen. How are you feeling?"

"My stomach is cramping, but I think my system is messed up."

"Last stool?"

"When I had the initial bleed. It nearly produced the baby."

"Shoot. We can't have you on the toilet then. Between gravity and pushing, you could have the baby right there. We'll have to figure something out."

"Prunes?" Mom offers.

"It's gonna take a lot more than prunes to get things moving without gravity," Eileen says. "I'm on again tomorrow, so we'll figure it out then. It could be an all-day project. We'll use a bedpan, and I'll pump you so full of laxatives you'll never know the difference."

I sigh and Eileen laughs. "There's no dignity in childbirth, Amy! Get over it!"

As soon as Eileen's back is turned, Mom fetches a bright yellow No Name package from the wardrobe and lops out a handful of prunes.

"Down the hatch," she orders. "No arguments. I know Eileen wants to fill you with laxatives, but a proper diet will help. Here, eat three now."

"They're so gross!" I complain, munching and swallowing hard.

"Don't whine. Here—three more. Tomorrow morning, we'll send Josh off to church and then we'll sort you out."

"Poop-day," I groan.

"It all comes down to the basics, as unglamorous as they are—eating, sleeping, pooping and, in your case, breathing."

"Like a baby." I smile.

"Like a baby."

At that moment, my baby gives a dramatic kick. Even covered by a nightgown, my stomach lurches as if the little person says, "I'm here, but be careful, Mom. No risk-taking. I'm still too wee to come."

• • •

SUNDAY MORNINGS IN MY CHILDHOOD WERE ALWAYS A SCRAMBLE. Dad did farm chores until the last possible moment, then showered in the grungy back bathroom. He would emerge in a suit laid out by Mom, his damp hair still fragrant with a lingering whiff of the barn. We had a long drive to church, a disadvantage of farm life, but were always on time for Sunday school or an even earlier choir rehearsal. With three girls in the house, mirror time was scheduled. Saturday ironing was encouraged. Sleeping in was not permitted.

This Sunday morning is much more leisurely than those of my childhood. Josh goes to church, and Mom and I read magazines, waiting for the stool softener I've guzzled to take effect.

"I don't know what to expect," I say. "Will I shoot off like a rocket and bump my head on the headboard?"

"I hardly think so." Mom rolls her eyes. "I'd count on a good stomach ache before production."

I flip through an article on spring fashion. Stripes and chevron patterns are in vogue. Peplums, those cheerful little flounces around the waist, are making a comeback. I'm in favour of all three, though not at the same time. Runway designers don't share my view.

"Did peplums do much for anybody's figure the last time they came around?" I ask Mom.

"You mean in the eighties?"

"Yeah, when we were kids, I think you had a dress or two with peplums."

"I was too short to pull them off, but they certainly were popular. They made us chubby girls look chubbier, which is never good fashion."

"Well, they're back."

"And I'm smart enough to avoid them."

"You're much skinnier now."

"Not that skinny."

Mom and I carry on so easily that a casual observer might guess I'm shooting the breeze with my mother while recovering from an appendectomy. In truth, I'm at significant risk of furthering the bulge of my membranes, perhaps even to the point of giving birth. But there is no getting away from it—I can't keep company with an impacted bowel forever. I decide to educate myself.

"Can I see the bedpan?" I ask.

"You've never seen a bedpan?" Mom replies incredulously.

"Why would I? I've never been on bed rest before."

"True." From a cupboard, Mom retrieves a grey plastic dish with a handle at one end and a tapered ridge on the other.

"You have got to be kidding me," I sputter. "How do you perch on that dustpan? Which end is which?"

"The flat end goes under you."

"Seriously? There has to be a better design than that. You could cut yourself on that weapon!"

"Yeah, well, this is the model you're going to perch on. Fracture bedpan…I think is the proper term."

I start to protest again but a cramp hits. I realize this process isn't going to be easy. I have a tsunami of angry sludge on the far side of an impacted bowel with only one path to the exit. My stomach feels like a battleground with canons loaded and fuses lit, foot soldiers marching in all directions, and arrows piercing the linings of every-thing. I'm in agony but, after an hour or two, Eileen is overjoyed with my progress.

"Don't try to push, Amy!" she says. "It will come with a boom and a bang. I've given you enough stuff to set a rocket on its way!"

It's past noon by the time the levee breaks and the dam explodes. It's a humiliating experience with Eileen cheering as if I'm producing triplets and Mom clucking, "Oh, how wonderful!" But by the time the last flush eradicates the evidence I'm still in one piece. The baby is still inside and no obvious damage has been done to the rather delicate arrangement of my nether region. My mother deserves a medal, if for no other reason than for putting up with all of my complaining; and I wouldn't be surprised if Eileen filed paperwork for early retirement. Delivering babies is one thing; delivering what she delivered today is quite another.

"You must be sorry you came," I say to Mom, apologetically.

"Don't be so dramatic. This had to be dealt with and you didn't want Josh around."

"But this is more than hot water bottle–running or pillow-fluffing. This is some serious child care."

"Nonsense. It's what mothers do. Look what you're doing for your child—bed rest, a catheter line, a seized-up back, fluid on the lungs, an official 'today's the day for pooping' day—and you haven't even got to labour yet. That's not exactly the mothering of the sto-rybooks, is it?"

"It's a crappy deal for sure," I mutter as Mom sinks into the easy chair. For once, she doesn't reprimand what she normally considers a vulgar adjective. Instead, she mutters, "Too true," ironically, and shuts her eyes for a nap.

Chapter 11

BY THE NEXT MORNING, I'VE BEEN IN HOSPITAL FOR FIVE DAYS and am no longer considered in danger of immediately giving birth or drowning in my own fluid-filled lungs. My bed is needed for more pressing cases, so my catheter and IV lines are removed, and I'm transferred down the hall to the Maternity unit, where I'll stay until the baby is born.

"Think of it as a change of scenery," Eileen suggests.

My new room looks west, over a medical helicopter landing pad. Large windows allow the late afternoon sun to shine over the two beds, which face each other. Down the middle of the room, a bright blue privacy curtain hangs on a hundred small chains. The other bed is vacant, but I'm warned a roommate will soon join me. There's no foldout chair-bed for a companion, just two heavy wooden chairs that vie with Muskoka deck chairs for weight and noise when dragged. The décor is hospital-bland, as if patients wouldn't be able to handle the excitement of real colour. African-violet-blue chair upholstery? No, indeed. A faded-sweater-grey will do. Bronzed brick façade? Best paint it over with a frail shade of insipid coral. The colour palette reminds me of a cheap print left hanging in sunshine for a decade or two.

Mom and Josh transfer my things from Labour and Delivery in a plus-size, super-wide wheelchair. Two browning bananas, a block of crumbling cheddar cheese in a Ziploc bag, and the inescapable sack of dried prunes all lie on a crumpled issue of *The Economist*, wedged between my faux-crocodile overnight bag and my salt-splattered winter boots. Mom chats encouragingly about everything—the state of the bananas, the size of the family kitchen—but it doesn't work. My tears come in a sniffle, then in a sob, and then in great gulps of ugly crying.

"What's wrong?" Mom takes my hand.

"I don't know," I say, turning my face from hers.

"Are you feeling low?" She uses her mother's favourite description for anyone not at their best.

"I don't want to be here anymore. I want to go home."

Josh hands me a Kleenex. "But this is a good thing, Babe. The longer you are here, the better it is for the baby!"

"I know. That's why I feel bad for feeling bad," I say with no logic, just tears.

"Darling Amy, I'm so proud of you. Nothing about this situation is what we planned, but it's still better than what it could have been five days ago at the Central. You are brave. You are patient. You are going to be fine." He kisses me and I feel guilty for fussing.

A nurse appears. Blonde, early thirties, she wears chunky, black-framed glasses over a bronzed complexion that can only be achieved in wintry Ottawa through patronage of the Supertan Suntan Centre or a lengthy time-share in Bermuda.

"I'm Celine," she says. "I am here to try to make everything as good as possible. I know things seem overwhelming right now, but you will survive!"

"It's not going to be as bad as I think?"

"I didn't say that. In fact, it's going to be twice as bad as you think. You'll run out of reading material; you'll get roommates you want to kill; and your back will ache worse than you ever thought possible, but you will survive. I've seen women lie flat on their backs for nine or ten weeks and then give birth to beautiful, healthy babies."

"Even women with cases like mine?"

"Anything is possible. From what I see on your chart, your membranes are still intact, which is great. If your membranes rupture, that will be a whole other story, but for now you have every chance of waiting this out."

"Okay." I wipe my eyes.

"All right, Sweetie!" cheers Celine. "You just hang in there while your membranes hang out and everything will be okay!"

I giggle, which seemed to be Celine's goal.

"Have you always worked in Maternity, Celine?" Mom asks, launching into her "get-to-know-the-nurses" routine.

"No, I started in Emergency, but I couldn't hack twelve hours of total panic, so I switched to Labour and Delivery, which was just as bad. Nearly lost my hearing with all the screaming, though it was worth it to see the births. There are so few miracles in a hospital, you know?"—Mom nods in polite agreement—"Surgeries, gall bladder attacks, cancer. All bad stuff. But births are amazing. Still, the stress was too much, so I transferred here to Maternity."

"Much less drama?"

"Much. Every now and again, there's a big exception. Last year, a woman was in for hypertension. I was on the night shift, and at three in the morning I heard her yelling from the bathroom. She was on the floor and the baby's head was emerging. Thankfully, I remembered something from Labour and Delivery, so I managed to catch the little monkey before he hit the bathroom floor—can you imagine? The whole time I was yelling, so another nurse came and we got mom and baby on a stretcher and down to L and D. There were some wide eyes at the nurses' station when we came around the corner with the little guy, sopping wet, on his mom's tummy, with his cord still attached!"

Celine seems to enjoy storytelling. Through her vivid descriptions, we picture her holding her breath and dashing into a tubercular patient's quarantine room with missing equipment; purposely tripping over the feet of a lazy father who treated her like a waitress, sending his ice water everywhere; and joyfully high-fiving a security guard who hauled away a patient's verbally abusive boyfriend. We listen with rapt attention. We've nowhere else to go and, frankly, the stories, as Celine recalls them, are enthralling.

"See, Amy?" Celine says. "You thought you were too sad to laugh but you're not. You'll need good humour to survive this, but I'm here. Mom's here. And hubby isn't going anywhere. You're not alone."

I don't feel alone, at least not until Josh and Mom dim the lights and leave for home. Then the loneliness begins.

I watch ice pellets pinging the window. A storm is moving in, a substantial, late-in-the-season storm, the kind that starts as rain, changes to ice, and finishes with clumps of wet, heavy snow falling from low, gloomy clouds.

Nimbostratus. That's what those clouds are called. The term pops to my mind, undoubtedly for the first time since a unit on meteorology in grade seven science. It's odd how the brain files things away for years on end, then spurts out data with a flourish.

What will I remember about this day, years from now? I wonder. My mother comforting me? My husband calming me? Will I remember heavy ward chairs being scraped across the floor? The melodrama of Nurse Celine's stories? Will I remember the loneliness?

The strange surroundings make me feel cut off from everything familiar. It's as if the sterile uniformity of hospitalization has reset me. I'm another faceless, taxpaying Canadian citizen with a right to health care, a right to lie in a bed, a right to be cared for. I feel far from home, not just the townhouse that I share with Josh, but also the farm where I grew up.

I think of how quickly childhood passed, one hot summer rushing headlong into another school year, year after year. The natural progression of life led me to this hospital bed. Leave home. Go to university. Get married. Have a baby. Why not? It's to be expected. Then why am I lying in hospital, waiting to give birth to a micro preemie, wondering what happened between learning how to ride a bike and prenatal bed rest? There was stuff in between, but it feels compressed, like an entire movie squeezed into vignettes for the trailer.

My thoughts are interrupted by a nurse turning on the overhead light and flinging the privacy curtain down its ceiling tracks, rattling the chains. A chair is dragged and thumped against a wall. There's anxious talking, all in French, during which nurses come and go. Someone uses the shared bathroom and slams the door upon both entering and exiting. The cupboard doors are banged and, after forty-five minutes of noise and confusion, the lights are turned out and peace is restored, though frantic whispers between my new roommate and her companion waft through the privacy curtain.

Although I didn't have much control over my environment before, the arrival of a roommate feels like a whole other level of intrusion. Now sleep is in danger and it's my only real means of escape.

When I was a child, my benevolent parents would trot us kids to the hospital to visit the sick and the aging, often one and the same. Not enjoying the outing in the slightest, we'd listen, stiff with boredom, as the conversation always turned to the same complaint: the patient wasn't getting any rest. I always wondered what they needed rest for. They weren't going anywhere or doing anything, so what was the big deal? But as I lie awake in the middle of the night, listening to the whispering from the neighbouring bed, I have an epiphany: it wasn't rest those poor souls were lacking; it was sleep. Life is unbearable without it. Pain bites worse. Anger management evaporates. Patience disintegrates. Those poor old souls from my childhood—all dead and gone now—they just wanted to shut their eyes and escape.

I cry a bit, not much, just enough to make me feel ashamed of myself. I'm carrying on as if the world has ended, and my roommate is having a bad time too. She probably spent the day in the Emergency ward and that couldn't have been fun. She probably hoped for a private room too.

The democratic nature of public health care dictates all patients must share rooms if the need arises, like it or not. Sharing requires patience though, and I will have to produce some, whether or not I'm in the mood. It's just the way things are.

• • •

NURSE CELINE WAKES ME EARLY. IT'S ONLY SEVEN O'CLOCK, BUT someone read my medical chart and booked me into the cardio clinic for a heart ultrasound.

"Nothing to worry about," Celine says. "It's just because you had an irregular heartbeat as a teenager. We want to be sure everything's fine before you go into labour."

Celine holds my contact dish for me and I fit the lenses onto my eyes. Once I see clearly, I stare out the window in disbelief. Ottawa has disappeared overnight. There's nothing. No helicopter launch pad. No parking lots or sidewalks. Nothing. Just whiteness.

"Did it storm all night?" I ask as Celine unlocks my bed's brakes.

"Almost, Girlfriend. Started as freezing rain. Traffic is a ginormous nightmare." Celine rolls back the privacy curtain to reveal a porter in a hospital-issued green smock and black cargo pants waiting in the hall. "Pierre will take you to Cardio and back. Don't run away from home, kids!"

Desperate for diversion, I ask Pierre about the roads.

"So bad, Madame. I tell you. So bad," he says as he pushes me down the hall. "I am behind a city bus. It creeps along—okay, no problem—but then it starts going down Bank Street sideways and I say to myself, 'Pierre! What are you doing? Go home! Back to bed!'"

I laugh appreciatively. "I'm sure it's slow all over. I heard it started as rain."

"It did. Last night, weatherman says, 'Last storm of the season, I promise.' Well, I promise you, Weatherman, if this isn't the last storm of the season, I'm moving to the Dominican."

Pierre pushes my bed to the elevators and thumbs the down arrow button. When the door opens, exhausted residents stagger out, clutching Styrofoam coffee cups. Dark rings line their eyes. Their limp lab coats only partly cover the creases of their baby-blue scrubs.

Pierre pushes me into the elevator, and I blink at my bleak reflection in unavoidable full-length mirrors. My eyes, wiped clean of makeup, disappear into my puffy face. My hair is matted against my head. My lips are cracked and scabbed.

The elevator sinks, groaning and squeaking to a stop on the second floor. Pierre pushes me out, into a gloomy hallway with only a few overhead lights turned on. Perhaps the person tasked with flicking the switches is currently stuck at some corner, waiting on a snowplough.

"Hello? Hello?" Pierre calls into an office. "I've got patient Amy Boyes."

"Leave her in the hall," answers a voice still low and croaky from the earliness of the hour. "Al is running behind so there's no point in you waiting."

Pierre pushes my bed against the wall and disappears with a wave and a carefree, "*Au revoir.*"

On the wall beside me, a brightly coloured chart, "Guidelines for Performing a Comprehensive Transeso-phageal Echocardiogram," is pinned to a corkboard. According to the chart, snaking a camera down a patient's throat is the first step to a comprehensive performance.

From that grim vision, I turn to watch the waiting room occupants at the other end of the hallway. They're all elderly Caucasian men and they calmly scan the pages of outdated *Economist, Time,* and *Maclean's* magazines through reading glasses as they stoically wait for their names to be called.

Their Scottish tweed caps and leather gloves lie on empty chairs, but their thick jackets remain zipped up in the chilly waiting room. Sensible winter shoes protrude from under the hems of neutral dress pants and several pairs of galoshes lie on a rubber mat like trout on the bottom of a canoe. Occasionally, one of the men glances my way with a sympathetic smile, but mostly they break from their reading only to check their watches and harrumph at the passing of time. Collectively, they're a demographic; individually, they're neighbours who shouldn't be shovelling snow, fathers with bad hearts, grandpas who won't slow down.

The elevator dings and another gurney is pushed down the hall. The patient sits, but her head droops forward. Her grey, frizzy hair shields her face and she gazes at her bruised arms as if they are new appendages. She rotates her bony wrists and flexes her dirty fingers, inspecting one side, then the other. She seems shocked by the psychedelic bruises that bloom around needle-sized sores like mosquito bites gone mad. I wonder why she's here and if it may already be too late to help her.

Just then, Al, the ultrasound technician, appears, apologizing to everyone for his tardiness—to the receptionist, to the other technicians, to a confused-looking man pushing a mop, though that may have been by accident. He wedges my stretcher into a dark ultrasound room and, upon closing the door and dimming the lights, very awkwardly explains how he'll move a small piece of cloth over my left breast while performing the ultrasound. I offer a verbal assent. After all, I am aware of the general location of my heart and understand he'll be in the neighbourhood.

Al snaps grainy pictures of my heart with an elaborate delicacy, tugging the little cloth a half inch here or there. I listen to the machine-amplified swish of blood pumping through my body. The sound reminds me of lifting the washing machine lid mid-cycle to pitch in a pair of socks. Privileged to the beast's mysterious workings, you can watch the water splash, soap suds froth, and wands lurch. Like the sound of my heart, churning out blood.

"This is a routine procedure," Al explains. "By the look of your chart, you've got better things to occupy your time."

"Ta," I say dryly, "but I have remarkably little to occupy my time at present."

Al turns off the machine and the swishing sound fades away. He pushes me back into the hall, which has all the lights turned on now. "Best wishes," he says, leaving me.

I anxiously wait for Pierre, as if this delay is keeping me from more pressing appointments. It's not as if I have a single thing I need to do today, so it's funny how habitual my impatience has become. Eventually Pierre saunters down the hall and recites, through coffee breath, the snowfall amounts for my benefit: "Twenty centimetres in Ottawa, a little less in the country. Last year, this time, it was beach weather. Can you believe it?"

I can believe it. This is Canada in March. Spring isn't guaranteed for a long time yet.

By the time I'm returned to my room, I am in high spirits. Getting out of my room did me a world of good, which reveals a lot about my mental state. Mom and Josh are waiting for me and they look absolutely frayed.

"Ninety minutes on the Queensway!" Mom exclaims, chucking her coat over the back of a chair. "You can't imagine how slowly traffic was moving. I was glad Josh was driving, not me."

"Forty-five accidents this morning," Josh reads from his Blackberry. "I'll let the morning traffic die down, then I'll go in to work. Is that all right with you?"

"Of course," I say. "I've got Mom. And don't worry—I'm in good form. I really enjoyed getting out this morning."

"Oh, wow." Mom rolls her eyes.

• • •

MY ROOMMATE, ACCORDING TO MOM'S SHARP EYES AND EARS, WEARS A hijab, is seven months pregnant, and has a blood clot. She's visited throughout the day by many concerned relations. They come, dragging chairs, gabbing loudly in French, laughing uproariously. Napping is impossible, so Mom and I play Scrabble, a game I normally excel at. But my best word is "liner," on a double letter for the "l." Six points. We decide our hearts aren't in it and call it a draw after a half hour.

Dad calls.

Grandma calls.

My sister Mavis calls.

We report the same non-news over and over again. The height of excitement occurs when the lunch cart arrives. Unfortunately, lunch is a packaged tuna sandwich shipped in from who-knows-where. At approximately 1:07 PM, I begin looking forward to the supper cart.

It's depressing to think my life has been reduced to anticipating the next food cart, but all the relaxation is driving me mad. It's unnerving. Wasteful. I'm not cut out for it. Relaxation is all well and good when you need it, but after a while you feel like an early contender for *My 600-lb Life*. I don't want to run a marathon, but getting up and washing my hair seems like a good idea.

"Just be glad you haven't gone into labour," Mom says for the millionth time.

I am glad, very glad, in fact, but I'd be more glad if someone came in and announced that my membranes were no longer hanging south of where they belong. But that isn't going to happen. I'm bleeding too badly to entertain wishful thinking.

And so Mom and I spend the day, saying the same things over and over again, buoying each other up with pleasantries, watching the clock for definite movement. When Mom leaves with Josh for the night, undoubtedly relieved to escape the hospital, the room is quiet on both sides of the curtain. I hope to drift off, if for no other reason than to kill the next eight hours with sleep.

But, just before midnight, my roommate's husband arrives. I surmise from the prolonged kissing and energetic chatter in French that he has previously been unavailable to visit. And though I understand their animation, I resent the noise. I want to sleep and they're keeping me awake.

They continue whispering breathily, frequently punctuating laughter with wet kisses. Then, sheets rustle and the bed creaks, so I hope he's hopped in with her with the intention of sleeping. But no such luck. Moans begin. Sighs. Little cries of pleasure. From what I can hear, the man is making out with his pregnant, blood-clotted wife in a shared hospital room. It's really too much.

"*Pardon*! SHHHHH! *Merci*!" I snap across the room.

My unkindness frightens me, but the pair aren't intimidated in the least. They continue as before, though possibly with louder moans.

My eyes burn with hot, salty tears. I want to be home, away from these loud, rude people, away from this democratic herding of strangers into collective bedrooms. I reach a box of Kleenex from the nightstand, and shred a tissue, stuffing the pieces into my ears. It makes no difference.

A light from the hallway slices through the room as the night nurse checks my roommate. When she leaves, I call to her and she replies with a soft—"Are you okay, Amy?"

"No. I'm not okay," I mutter. "I want to sleep and my roommates are loud. Could you ask them to be quiet? It's after midnight!"

"They are in bed so I'm sure they'll be sleeping soon," she says conciliatorily, then dashes out of the room before I can protest further. Even before the door clicks shut, the pair across the curtain are at it again, kissing and moaning.

I realize the nurse doesn't want to referee, and it can't be easy to judge between one patient's right to see her husband and another patient's right to a quiet environment, but someone has to be in charge. The night nurse is as good a candidate as any.

I briefly consider calling 911. Wouldn't that show the night nurse? It would be fun to have a paramedic run up to the Maternity ward. If only I could convince them I was having a nervous breakdown. Shouldn't be too hard. The 911 dispatcher might not respect a call originating from a hospital bedside phone though.

I decide to count the night as a write-off and begin plotting retribution for the morning: Mom will demand I be moved to a private room and, if refused, then Josh will see how much a private room costs to book. I'll talk to the day nurse and explain the difficulties. Maybe I'll be lucky and the day nurse will be Celine. She'll understand. She'll see I'm losing my mind and she'll care, not like this night nurse who won't demand anything from anyone. Coward!

My plotting gets less coherent and stops making any sense, even by my own crazed standards. I'm aware of noise from the other side of the blue curtain, but black clouds shadow my thinking. My eyelids are too heavy to keep open, even for a moment.

Chapter 12

PAIN WAKES ME. LOW IN MY ABDOMEN, A CLENCHING INCREASES until it reaches some invisible ceiling, then slithers away. I lie still and wait for nothing more to happen. But more pain comes and it's terribly sad because, despite all the labour scares of the past week, I have a panicked suspicion this could be it. This pain feels like it knows what it's doing.

Getting up no longer feels like a crime, so I flip back the bed sheets and shuffle to the shared bathroom, holding the door open longer than necessary to illuminate both sides of the room before letting it slam shut. I want my roommates to wake. I want them to suffer as I have suffered.

In the bathroom, my suspicions are confirmed: I am bleeding profusely. Fresh ketchup blood, amniotic fluid, old bronzed clumps—it's all there, flowing out of me. My nightgown is stained. My legs are streaked. I know I shouldn't be walking, but since it probably doesn't matter anymore, I inch my way out of the bathroom, out of the hospital room, into the bright hall.

"Nurse?" I call hesitantly, blinking at the blurry nurses' station.

My nurse hops up from behind the high counter. "Amy! What are you doing out of bed?"

"I'm badly bleeding and I'm in pain," I say without much emotion. I'm too tired to express all the fear and frustration that I feel. I just hope she'll do more about this complaint than she did my last one.

"To bed! Right now," she orders, leading me back. To my distracted satisfaction, she makes a lot of noise as she turns on lights, hauls in machines, and fastens a contraction monitor around my midsection. As another pain begins, I cry out louder than is necessary and am rewarded with the sound of my roommates stirring.

The night nurse crouches in front of the contraction monitor, her eyes level with the screen. "Yeah…" she says, her voice trailing off as a line descends from a spiky Everest-shape. "That's a contraction for sure. You're going back to Labour and Delivery."

"Is this labour?"

"I don't know and we're not chancing it. You need to be next to the NICU in case the baby comes."

She scoops up my purse and laptop and piles them on my bed beside my legs—"Someone can come back for the rest of your stuff in the morning." She unlocks the bed's brakes, lines the bed up with door, and shoves. Just like that, I'm out of the miserable room, away from the strangers. I'm rushed down a windowless hallway, past half-empty food carts, past two automatic doors that swing open in front of us. I'm back in the depths of the hospital now, back in Labour and Delivery. It could well be the only ward where results are either celebrated or buried. There's no in between.

• • •

THERE'S A MOMENT SOMEWHERE AROUND SEVEN O'CLOCK THE next morning when I realize time is skipping along and, since time has not skipped along for the rest of my hospital stay, I assume I'm slightly out of my head.

There's no timeline for the day, no schedule of events, just a hodge-podge of impressions. People in. People out. Pains come. Pains go.

Mom documents my contractions with a stubby pencil on the back of a grocery list she found at the bottom of her purse. Under oranges and ham, my contractions are listed: 6:48, 7:01, 7:10. Mom sits beside me patiently, not seeming to mind the hard chair or lack of food or drink. It's labour day and she's here for the duration.

Josh paces from the window to the chair, then back again. He hasn't shaved, so a dark smudge of stubble clouds his face. He bites his lip and jams his hands into his pant pockets as he paces.

At half-past seven, the shift changes and Nurse Eileen arrives, exuding Caribbean cheerfulness.

"What are you doing in here, kid?" she teases. "You are supposed to be taking it easy over in Maternity!"

I smile weakly. "Couldn't stay away."

"That's all right. I feel special. You're booked for an ultrasound at eight o'clock, so the porter should be here shortly. I can see your contraction monitor from the nurses' station, so that's where I'll be. I'll be back when the porter arrives."

At eight o'clock, Eileen storms back into my room snapping, "Well, I don't know where that idiot porter is, so I'll take you myself. I'm not going to call to cancel him either. He can take a walk up here for all I care!"

We all go—me flat on my back on my labour bed, Mom trotting alongside, Josh pushing the bed with Eileen. They wheel me into the ultrasound room and I know what to expect. The darkness, the grainy, grey blobs—it feels like a routine now, a ritual to be performed.

A contraction begins, so the technician rushes to get the wand on my stomach before it ends. She watches the screen with a strange look on her face, then moves the wand between my legs to view the baby from below.

I watch the ceiling monitor and wonder what I'm seeing. A dark black circle (presumably the birth canal) fills the screen, and during contractions a bit of white throbs in and out of it. As another contraction begins, the picture clears and I see what is throbbing. It's a little foot kicking into the birth canal.

The technician watches, wincing. "Rest here a minute, okay, Amy?" she says in a high, cheerful voice. "I'll be right back."

She scurries out of the room and returns a minute later with Eileen.

"We're going to get you back in your room, Amy," Eileen says casually, too casually, like a police officer trying to shoo a crowd away from an accident scene—"Nothing to see here. Off you go. That's it."

We return to my room and, as soon as the bed brakes are locked and the contraction monitor and fetal heart monitor are returned to my belly, Eileen takes a deep breath. "Honey-pie," she says, "your baby is kicking right into your birth canal. The baby is breeched and it's coming soon."

"How soon?"

"Within hours."

Her words land like punches, big sledgehammer swings to all my hopes.

"I know, Sugar." Eileen touches my hand. "You kept hoping this wasn't the real deal, but this baby of yours is tumbling right on out. And there's more: the lab results are in and your membranes are infected. The baby has to come now because the infection could travel and then we're all in big trouble. So right now, I'm going to get a resident to assess you and then you're going to get to work."

Eileen runs from the room, leaving us in various states of shock. Mom blinks rapidly, trying not to cry, though not very successfully. Josh nods robotically, staring into nothing.

"All of this hoping and praying, yet here we are," I whisper. "This is happening."

I grip Mom's fingers as another pain hits, but I'm losing energy. I have no drive to get on with labour because I also want the baby to stay inside. It's a counter-intuitive process. I want the pain to end, just not in childbirth, sixteen weeks early. It isn't what we planned. I was going to lie here for weeks and weeks like all those women in the stories. But I've only managed seven days. Just seven.

Mom and Josh pat whatever part of my body is within their easy reach, then return to their earlier posts: Mom charting contractions, Josh rubbing my feet and pacing. I lie back on knotted hair and squint up at the water-stained ceiling panel. I'm not humoured by the koala anymore though. It's just a dirty ceiling tile, ill-fitting in the grid. I don't understand why such a disgusting ceiling is allowed in a labour room. Doesn't anybody care what women look at during the longest days of their lives?

• • •

MORNING FADES INTO AFTERNOON AND AFTERNOON INTO EARLY evening as pains come closer together. I no longer have time to rest between them; the head of one attaches itself to the tail of another.

I want it to stop but, like every mother in the history of the world, I realize once labour begins, there's no escape chute, no alternative way to spend the day.

After a few hours, Eileen brings a gas mask and I grasp it over my face when the pains come. I try to breathe like Eileen coaches, but my head swings from side to side all on its own.

"Breathe, Amy. Just breathe." Mom speaks with authority, as if breathing were an actual possibility. When my back arches from the pain, she gently pushes down my shoulder. "No, Amy. That's not going to help. You need to breathe."

A neonatologist comes to discuss resuscitation drugs with Josh and they stand at the foot of my bed, the doctor with his binders, Josh with a million questions. Term after term, factoid after factoid, the doctor's painstakingly detailed descriptions prompt Josh to ask questions of increasing minutiae. I don't want to hear it all again—the stages of lung development, the chances of labour-induced mortality, the odds of brain damage. My irritation is likely exaggerated by labour pains, but in the middle of a contraction I kick Josh's leg and point to the door. He takes the hint and the two disappear to the hallway.

Then it gets dark. Gloomy. Lights are turned on, but no one suggests supper.

I refused an epidural early in the afternoon but now I want it because the pains are bad. Like snakes suffocating their prey, they circle my abdomen, cut off my breath and sicken my stomach. Just when I think, "Ah, yes, this is the top, this is the worst," the pains intensify. I wonder how bad they'll get before it's over. The contractions feel like fire ripping through me. The baby is tiny. Why am I suffering so much?

"Please, Eileen," I whisper. "I'm tired—can I have an epidural?"

Eileen nods. "You got it. We'll fix you up."

A spectacled anaesthesiologist arrives a few minutes later. She looks about twenty-two though she has to be much older to be an anaesthesiologist. She's dressed in operating room garb—blue scrubs, bright plastic shoe covers, a surgical cap. She looks kind, sympathetic even.

"I usually have patients sit up and squeeze into a tight ball," she says, "but because we're trying to avoid pressure on the baby, I'll have you roll onto your side and arch your back instead. It's trickier but I can make it work. There are risks with every procedure, including the possibility of spinal damage and of a massive headache," she goes on, scanning my medical charts. "I'll be able to tell you after the injection whether or not you'll have the headache."

"It's okay. Do it." I squeeze Mom's hand harder. Another pain has begun.

"We'll wait for this contraction to end," the anesthesiologist says, "then we'll go quickly because you can't move while I am inserting the needle. We'll try to catch you between contractions."

The room falls silent as the anaesthesiologist and Eileen watch the monitor. The contraction traces upwards and then, as it begins to lose momentum, they snap into action, Eileen easing me onto my right side, directing my head low against my chest, the anaesthesiologist tearing a six-inch epidural puncture needle from its sterile packaging. Eileen pulls my knees up, pats my hip comfortingly, then unknots the ties of my nightgown. The massive, bloody pad that lies underneath me slides off to one side, but no one seems to care; stained sheets don't matter at this stage.

Mom strokes my hair and Josh crouches beside me holding my cold hands in his. As Eileen washes my back with antiseptic, I shut my eyes and hold my breath.

It only lasts a minute: the icy swab, the massive pressure, the odd sense of numbness. Soon, the pain evaporates and I'm free. Compared to labour, the epidural is pure heaven. Nothingness replaces the agony of the past sixteen hours.

"Thank you," I whisper to the anaesthesiologist as Eileen returns me to my back.

"You won't have a headache," she says, gathering her equipment. "I can tell you that for sure." She strokes my hand—"Best luck to you"—then leaves with Eileen.

Mom turns off the overhead lights and pats Josh's shoulder. "Try and rest," she says.

Josh curls up in the easy chair, and Mom returns to her chair beside my bed, resting her elbows on my mattress, her chin in her palms. As the daylight fades behind the window blinds, her eyes grow heavy, their wrinkles deepening into shadow-filled crevices.

"You okay, Mom?" I whisper.

"Of course, Sugar Plum. You should sleep though. The epidural won't last forever and you might have a long night ahead of you."

"I love you, Mom. You know that, don't you?"

"Of course. Sleep now, Amy."

I close my eyes, but my repose is short-lived. As I'm drifting off, Dr. Ahmed bursts in, flicking on lights, weaving a portable ultrasound machine around the chairs in his way.

"No, no, Amy," he says, "I need to see the baby before you sleep."

He searches for an electrical plug-in on the wall behind me, then powers on the machine. After spreading gel over the ultrasound wand, he presses the wand against my belly button. Using slow, careful circles, he moves the wand lower and lower until it's between my legs. Then he sighs a tired sigh and flicks off the machine with a loud click.

"The baby is breeched and is completely in the birth canal except for its head," he snaps. "It has to be born right now. Eileen! Get the NICU nurse in here and alert the resuscitation team. Turn on all the lights! Amy, do you understand? You have to have the baby now!"

And that's it. I'm having a baby sixteen weeks early and there's no stopping it.

● ● ●

SOMEONE SAYS I NEED TO PUSH BUT, FLOATING AS I AM ON AN EPIDURAL, I don't know when I'm contracting.

"I'll watch for you, Sweetheart," Eileen says, her eyes on the contraction monitor. She drums her fingers on the top of the monitor, then calls, "Now, Amy! Now!"

I push and Eileen cheers, so I assume I have the hang of it, but frankly I have no idea what I'm doing. I can't feel below my waist, so

I'm mostly imitating anything I've seen on *Call the Midwife*, Season 1. There's likely more technique involved than what can be shown at eight p.m. on the BBC, but I didn't make my prenatal classes, so I fly blind.

In the moments between contractions, I notice my own nakedness. When I was in pain, I didn't care who saw what, but now that the epidural has taken effect I'm mentally free to consider the great swath of skin lying before me and the gathering of people surveying it. Mom clasps my right knee; Eileen, my left. Josh practically hovers over the action zone, anxious to see the first sign of the little person. Around the end of the bed, two residents, Dr. Ahmed, and the nurse who will run the baby down the hall to the Neonatology Intensive Care Unit all stand ready.

One of the residents wears a pair of protective glasses—"for splashes"—and in their reflection, I watch the most marvellous sight. As I push, a sac emerges. It looks like a freezer bag bulging with mashed beets. With each push, the sac stretches and blossoms into a sphere, balanced perfectly between my legs. When it grows to the size and shape of an overripe beefsteak tomato, almost translucent from the heat of summer, the doctor pokes it with a hooked stick, and it slips away with a splash.

And there she is. Under my left leg lies the smallest baby I've ever seen. She's a tiny clump of crimson wrinkles that could easily fit within my two hands. She makes wobbly protestations and flails scrawny, liquorice-like limbs in the air. Dr. Ahmed dashes her off the sticky sheet and snips the umbilical cord, the last link between us. He hands her to the NICU nurse and she pounds out the door to the waiting resuscitation team. Josh follows with the camera bouncing around his neck.

And that's it. It's all over—the wait, the uncertainty, the pain. After a week of panic and boredom and fear, it's all over. And I don't cry, not one tear. I'm just happy to no longer be responsible for keeping my baby alive. It's someone else's job now, someone who knows what they're doing, not me.

There's a triumphant buzz in the room as the umbilical cord is packaged and labelled, the ultrasound machine wheeled back out to the hall, and the contraction monitor unsnapped and put away. The labour is everyone's success, and perhaps the Labour and Delivery team is also relieved to no longer be responsible for the baby's welfare. Leave it to the neonatologists. They're the experts.

One by one, the room empties until suddenly it's just Eileen and Mom, rolling up blood-soaked sheets, bathing me with wet cloths, sliding a fresh nightgown over my head.

"Well done, Sugar-Pie," Mom says. "I'm so proud of you!"

"She came out crying!" I gush. "She has to be breathing if she was crying!"

"Sure, Honey, sure," Eileen soothes.

A few minutes later, Josh dashes back into my room, his eyes radiant, his smile euphoric.

"The heart is strong and they've got her breathing on the ventilator!" he blurts. "She's one pound, six ounces though—quite small."

I motion to the camera around his neck. "Show me."

He holds the back of the camera toward me so I can see the pictures he's taken. On the LCD monitor, I see Madeline lying in the middle of a resuscitation table. She's positioned spread-eagle while the resuscitation team reach from outside the picture's frame, inserting a ventilator tube down her throat and an IV line into her arm. Her chest is covered in circular sensors and something that looks like a teabag is fastened to her clipped umbilical cord. She lies in a Ziploc bag—a medium freezer size, perhaps. Josh explains that the plastic bag will keep her skin hydrated during the resuscitation. A warming lamp glows over her as the resuscitation team scurries to stabilize her in this unbelievable new environment. Her lungs, never intended to function at twenty-four weeks, must begin to absorb air. Her heart, beating so faithfully through labour, has to patter under the huge strain. Her bowel and intestinal system must begin processes they're wholly unprepared for. And her brain, her poor little brain, has to cope with an onslaught of stimuli: light, noise, scent, the sensation of a ventilator tube, the pain of an IV line.

I push away the camera. "Go back, Josh. Be with her."

He leaves, and I don't feel as comforted by the pictures as I thought I would be. Madeline's survival already requires much intervention. I can see that for myself. I had optimistically hoped that despite the long odds everything would work out easily enough. But now I feel a deep-seated panic, the same one I felt when they told me horrible things about membranes. I suspect we're about to live the worst days of our lives.

Chapter 13

DR. FIALA, A NEONATOLOGIST, LOOKS HARD AT JOSH AND ME AND asks, "Do you understand the situation?"

She waits for some reaction, so we nod. It feels like the thing to do.

"I'm not sure what more I can tell you," she continues. "At twenty-four weeks gestation, sixteen weeks premature, Madeline will be lucky to survive this week. Yes, the resuscitation was successful, but infections are common at this stage. Although she seems strong, she's still within the first seventy-two hours. After that, breathing will be our biggest problem because her lungs are underdeveloped. Frankly, her lungs are hardly even formed and, without fully developed sacs, she doesn't absorb oxygen effectively. Picture a cactus in the desert—that's what Madeline's lungs are like. They soak up moisture and hold it, making it impossible for her to breathe on her own."

"Her lungs will fill with fluid and she'll tire out. Is that what you're saying?" Josh asks, his voice almost shaking.

"Oh, she'll definitely exhaust herself, and that's not a problem in and of itself—we can always turn up the oxygen flow in the ventilator—but, if an infection takes hold, she'll have no reserves to fight it. We have powerful antibiotics but they can only do so much."

"Is she in pain, do you think?" I whisper.

"Most likely. We have her on a sedative to keep her quiet, so that will help with any discomfort she might be feeling. We are feeding her small amounts of milk, but her bowels are underdeveloped, so there's a good chance they'll block or perforate. If that happens, she'll certainly be in pain, but we'll deal with that if we have to."

The doctor looks away and I feel alone. It doesn't matter how much love and support comes from family and friends. At the end of the day, it's still just the two of us, sitting across from the doctor, listening to horrendous things, wishing it was all over.

And friends have been encouraging, almost to the point of absurdity. I've heard endless stories about dear old granddads who were born sixteen weeks early in a cabin due west of Pakenham and survived handily, growing up to be lumbermen. But I doubt their great-grannies' math. They couldn't have been sixteen weeks premature. Dr. Fiala is describing a long, painstaking hospitalization, filled with interventions and complications. I don't think any twenty-four week preemie could survive without optimal care, or at the very least a ventilator.

"What about her other organs? Heart? Brain?" Josh forms his words cautiously, as if Madeline's well-being depends on the precision of his speech.

"Her heart ultrasound this morning showed a murmur, but that's to be expected," the doctor replies. "It's just a hole between the pulmonary artery and the aorta. Instead of healing at birth like it would in a full-term baby, it remains open, contributing to low blood oxygen saturation, weight loss, and lethargy. The condition may heal on its own, or we may need to treat it through medication or surgery. We can wait and see. Now, brain wise—she'll have a scan in a week to check for bleeds."

"Bleeds?" I ask, arching my eyebrows.

"Just as they sound—haemorrhages of the brain's fragile blood vessels caused by the stress of premature birth. They are quite common among the severely premature and they vary in severity. Madeline will be checked once a month for the duration of her hospitalization, but if she is to have bleeds they will likely happen in the first week."

"And if she has them?" Josh asks.

"There's not much we can do. She'll be followed closely until she is a toddler to watch for intellectual and physical disabilities."

Disabilities. I suck in my breath. I had somehow hoped we'd get off easily, but now I picture wheelchairs, ramps, computer-assisted communication devices, portable oxygen tanks...

"If she survives," I say, choking through my words, "how long will she be in hospital?"

"Oh, I can't say," says Dr. Fiala. "Every baby is different. Some go home before their due dates, some quite a bit after. You need to get through this first week, then brace yourself for a sixteen-week stay, which," she adds in a hush, "is the very best-case scenario. However, I paint a dismal picture because I want you to brace yourselves. But it's okay to hope too. We just have to wait to see what Madeline's journey will be. In the meantime, prepare yourselves for anything. It's best this way."

We look at our hands, at our shoes, at the tiled floor, anywhere but at Dr. Fiala. We don't want to face the ugly truth presented by the kind and gentle doctor. It's the combination of message and messenger that jars us. If the dire news had come in a stapled report, we'd be braced for its severity, but this way—whispered sympathetically by another mother—confuses our expectations. Nice people don't tell you horrible things. They just don't.

"Any more questions?" the doctor asks.

We shake our heads, so she leaves us alone, sitting bolt upright on the sagging couch, like fence posts rammed into shifting clay. We're hardly aware of each other's presence, yet we hold hands, my left in Josh's right. He grips my hand so tightly that my rings dig into my fingers. We feel each other's anxiety, our stress, but we don't comfort each other. We just stare numbly into dusty corners as intercoms and alarms sweep over us.

"She looks so fragile," I murmur.

"I know." Josh closes his eyes, inhaling deeply, perhaps trying to free himself from the fear that grips his chest. He hasn't slept decently in a week and looks it. His eyes are smudged dark. His hair is matted and greasy. I know I look the same but I don't care. In fact, I care about so little it frightens me. All the things that worried me last week have faded away—income tax filing, studio scheduling, meals in the freezer—wisps of smoke, nothing more.

Josh and I finally look at each other—husband, wife; father, mother—but we don't smile, not even a forced smile of reassuring optimism. It would take too much energy; besides, we understand how the other feels. We're stunned by what we've seen and heard. We've glimpsed the dark side of nature, its capability to churn out mistakes, to mangle lives, and it happened too quickly to make sense of it. Yet, we must pull ourselves together. My room in the Maternity Ward must be packed up and my discharge papers signed. Groceries have to be bought and laundry has to be washed. There is a life to return to even if we don't remember it. We pull ourselves off the couch and tiptoe to Room A for one more look at Madeline.

She lies on her back in an incubator, a limp bundle of wrinkled flesh, taped and wired to multiple lines. She has no will of her own, no strength. Her survival relies on the array of machines around her incubator, tallying up numbers and percentages, pumping oxygen and nutrients into her body through narrow lines.

The incubator's thick, curved Plexiglas walls bend our perception, like a glass of water confusing the world beyond. Although the incubator protects and warms her, it also keeps us away. We are outsiders, observers. Look, but don't touch.

A quilt, sewn by a volunteer, covers the incubator, blocking sunshine by day and fluorescent light by night. Lifting the corner of the quilt feels like a sacred ritual, a prayer in action. I lift, look, and breathe, "Oh dear God. She looks so awful. So very, very awful. Save her, I pray. Save her."

As each hour since birth slides by, I begin to accept her death as inevitable. I hadn't pictured a loss after birth, but that's what it will be—a labour-in-vain, a miscarriage, a "not-meant-to-be," as people so infuriatingly say. I always thought if I were to lose a baby, it would happen early on, at twelve weeks maybe, a splash of blood and then—all over. But a birth, followed by a suffering death, might be the cruellest loss of all. I will have to watch her give up. At least if I had miscarried, I wouldn't have to see her fingers claw when needles are sunk into her veins, or listen to the alarms wail when her oxygenation plummets and heart rate drops down to nothing.

Through the gap in the incubator's blanket, I memorize Madeline's face in case she gives up before I return later this evening. It's an odd face, barely formed. So impossible. So strange to see.

A ghastly memory flashes and I try to ignore it, but it won't go away. It keeps coming back to mind, to the mental view that flits away when you really try to look at the details. It's from when I was a little girl on the farm. I was six or seven maybe, visiting a batch of new baby piglets in the farrowing barn. Outside their pen though, Dad had piled a half-dozen stillborn piglets. Wet and red, awaiting burial, they were a mass of taut, translucent skin. They were haphazardly stacked because, really, they didn't matter anymore. They were dead.

The resemblance between those pigs and Madeline is uncanny. The wet, red skin. The fused eyes. The half-formed features. I want to gag, yet I can't turn away from the incubator. How can I? This poor child is mine.

As I watch Madeline, Josh peppers the nurses with questions: How does the rate of ventilation relate to her own breathing? Is she breathing above the ventilator at all? Why is her heart rate line tracing so irregularly on the monitor? What is in her IV?

He seems to absorb the nurses' answers, while to me, they fall like dust particles from the ceiling vent. The more I listen, the less I comprehend. I can't take in any new information because I still haven't accepted Madeline's birth as reality. I'm in denial.

I shuffle to a rocking chair and close my eyes, but when Josh is ready to go I don't want to leave. I slip back to the incubator for another look, but Josh tugs my arm. "Come on, Darling," he says. "We'll be back tonight."

I know we'll be back, in a matter of hours, but I still feel like we're abandoning our child, leaving her in the care of strangers, relinquishing our rights and responsibilities. Walking away feels unnatural, but there's nothing else to do. We are as helpless as she and are of no use to the nurses.

So we go home, praying there will be no official phone call, no sympathetic voice, no quiet entreaty to return as quickly as possible.

Chapter 14

MARCH IN OTTAWA IS OFTEN WINTRY AND THIS MARCH IS NO EX-
ception. Admitted to hospital wearing thick, woolly clothes, I still
need their warmth for discharge ten days later.

As I prepare go home, I slowly layer on tights, scarf, wool coat,
mittens. Getting dressed for the outside world feels like I'm admit-
ting nothing is wrong with me, that I'm not a patient anymore. But
I'm not well. My head throbs and my stomach churns. I feel like I'm in
a trance. A psychologist would probably diagnosis it as postpartum
depression. All very reasonable, of course, but I need to be brave for
Josh's sake and I don't want to be. I want to be coddled and cared for
and fussed over and that seems rather selfish with Madeline fighting
for her life.

I pack the last of my things and follow Josh and Mom into an
elevator that sinks away from the NICU, into the abyss of normal life.
On the ground level, the doors open and we stand back while the
elderly inch their way on and off the elevator. We dodge a mother
turning a baby stroller, then step around a man with a leg cast as
he propels his wheelchair across the crowded lobby. I envy the simplicity of his pain. What is a broken leg? It will heal. His life will be
normal again.

We step outside the hospital, and I wince against bright sunshine
on fresh snow. I fumble through my purse for my sunglasses, irritated.
It's as if the sun is shining just to show me how cross I am. But I
have a right to be cross, I tell myself. Nothing about today is what I
pictured. I'm leaving the hospital after having a baby, but Josh isn't
carrying a car seat with a blanket draped over it; Mom isn't wrest-
ling massive "Congratulations" balloons through doorways; I'm not
hauling a diaper bag. Instead we trudge through salty puddles to the
parking garage where Josh parked our car high on the third level.

Bags hang off our arms, heavy with many things that accumulated during my hospital stay.

Like a caravan of pack animals, we climb the crumbling parkade staircase slowly. Paint flakes off the metal handrails and bits of garbage litter the steps. I glare at the grunge-packed corners and feel increasingly exhausted with each step. I haven't had any exercise to speak of in the past ten days so my body rebels against moving. My legs shake and my breathing is ragged.

"Take your time," Mom says, so I stop to rest for a moment, then exhale at the low, dirty ceiling, and stomp on, right up to the third floor.

At the car, Josh unlocks the doors and we unload our burdens into the trunk: a bag of Macintosh apples, a pair of my ballet flats for the hospital hallways, a rented breast pump, my overnight bag with the bag of dried prunes tucked in an outside pocket. Josh slams the trunk lid, and the thump echoes off the low concrete ceiling like a clap of thunder on a muggy night. We climb in, Josh and I in the front, Mom in the back.

"Have enough room?"

"Fine, thanks."

Josh backs the car out of the narrow parking space, around the parkade's sharp corners, down the sloped driveway to the exit. He inserts a two-week parking pass into the box, and the barrier arms lift. His cautious frugality annoys me. If he had purchased the maximum four-week parking pass, I would feel that he had hope for a long hospital stay.

I stare dully out the window, but everything I see reminds me of my own misfortune. The number of women pushing strollers seems to have skyrocketed and everywhere I look there are minivans with their pointless "Baby On Board" sticker. Swing sets peek over backyard fences and tree houses perch in the broad branches of maples. I imagine all the houses are filled with happy children sleeping in beds, not incubators.

We drive past Ikea. A massive banner on the north wall advertises cribs. I wonder if we can still return ours. I may have junked the receipt.

"I moved all the baby things to the nursery and shut the door," Josh says quietly.

"Everything?" I press. "The name book, the stuffed animals, everything?"

"Yes. Everything."

I nod, satisfied. I'd rather keep our house neutral, one place where I'm not constantly reminded of the disaster.

I must doze off, for soon we are home. The house looks the same—a brown brick three-storey townhouse. A spring wreath hangs on the front door. Early bulbs peek out of a receding snowbank. Pine boughs from Christmas drop needles across the narrow porch. There's no evidence that the house's mistress fled in a panic last week.

I look around and am relieved not to see any neighbours. I don't have the energy to formulate an explanation for what's happened. We have to come up with an appropriate response to inquiries soon though—emails and phone calls from concerned friends and family arrive almost constantly—but it's hard to know what tone to take, what attitude to assume. Should we speak in a funereal hush about the improbability of survival? That may be melodramatic, as there's a chance that Madeline will survive; other twenty-four-week babies have. Or should we speak with ambiguous optimism about making the best of life's unpredictability? That feels more appropriate for a flooded basement or dented car fender, not for a life-or-death scenario.

I'm too tired to work it out now, so I walk quickly into the house and breathe a sigh of relief when the door clicks shut behind us. I can hear Michael teaching down the hall in the piano studio, so I take off my coat and boots quietly in order to avoid conversation.

We tramp up the stairs to the second level and pile all our bags and boxes onto the middle of the dining room floor, like the worldly goods of a refugee family heaped up in the middle of a train station rotunda. Mom has straightened the house, so there's no sign of the disaster but, like a crime scene after the cleaning crew's been through, the house seems artificial, hygienic, staged for resale. It's quiet though, a pleasant change from the bedlam of the hospital.

"I'm done," I sigh.

"Go for a nap," Mom says.

I climb another flight of stairs to our bedroom and shed my clothes into a heap in the middle of the floor. Removing the clothes I wore at the hospital feels like a cleansing process, a way to rid myself of the memories, the smells. I find a soft nightgown in my chaotic underwear drawer and tug it over my oddly shaped body, but it pulls unattractively over with my squishy stomach like cling wrap over play dough. Disgusted, I fish a big throw-sweater out of the pile of clothes on the floor and pull it over the worst of my bulges and rolls.

The sheets on my side of the bed are still snugly tucked between the mattresses, so I tug them loose, dragging them over my shoulders, inhaling their faint scent—a little laundry soap, a little Josh. It feels good to be back in my own bed, on my own terms. Bed rest in hospital quickly turned into a prison sentence—flat on my back, head below feet, blood rushing, back throbbing. A rest is supposed to be a pleasant thing but, like nearly all good things in life, it turned sour in excess.

At the foot of our bed, a canvas print hangs on the wall. It's of Josh and me on our wedding day, smiling blissfully. We look so much happier than we are now.

We were married just after Christmas, close to my parents' farm in Manitoba. A winter wedding is risky in most places, but on the prairies it was downright rash. During the dinner, or supper, as they say in the country, a blizzard began. We didn't want to miss our morning flight to Maui, so we left early for Winnipeg.

On drifted roads, through some of Canada's flattest farmland, we crept between snow-filled ditches and dark, wind-blown fields, and eyed the power lines to keep us straight. After two interminable hours, we crunched to a stop in axle-deep snow and stamped into the glowing rotunda of the Fort Garry Hotel. A towering Christmas tree twinkled, welcoming us from the miserable night, and beguiling piano riffs wafted in from the Palm Lounge. It was as if the hotel had remained open since 1913 just to greet us on our wedding night.

We were so happy, but all that feels long ago. Our wedding day has faded into silence like the shimmery upper-register piano licks. It was one day out of our lives, and now whatever happens to Madeline will colour every other day. She's changed everything.

We knew a baby would change our lives. I had heard enough from my older sisters to know parenting wasn't easy—"You can't even imagine how much poop there was, dripping out of his pants and down the side of the restaurant high chair!" or "We'd love to visit you, but there isn't money and travelling with kids is miserable"—but we never imagined this.

We imagined a healthy, happy child to love, for the pure joy of it. We wanted to take a pudgy hand in ours and explore the world together, revelling in all its peculiarities. We never pictured it being this difficult.

I think of my walks down the Katimavik footpath last summer. I was so worried about being a parent that I didn't think of how devastating it would be to not be one. My vision was narrow. I didn't understand that parenting is not about whether or not you're good enough or responsible enough to have a child. Parenting is about how a child changes you in a million different ways. It's about realizing your own convenience is secondary to the child's well-being; your own plans, inconsequential.

It seems to me though, as I close my eyes and try to sleep, that everything will blow up in our faces, and we'll be left with the haunting memory of standing over an incubator, feeling so terribly guilty.

• • •

"AMY! IT'S THE PHONE."

I wake to Mom gently shaking my shoulder with one hand, cupping the cordless phone with the other.

"Who is it?" I ask, annoyed.

"The public health nurse."

"Oh, for crying out loud."

I pull myself into a sitting position and flip back the sheets. I had been sleeping so soundly I hadn't heard the phone ring on the nightstand.

"Hello," I croak.

"Hi! I'm calling from the Healthy Babies Healthy Children Program," a woman says cheerfully. "Is this a good time for a chat?"

"Sure. It's okay."

"Great! I'm making contact to insure you receive all the information and support you need in the coming days. I have some questions that will help determine your physical and mental health as well as your infant's feeding and nutritional needs. First of all, allow me to offer my congratulations on the birth of...um..."

I hear pages rustling.

"...Madeline."

"Are you aware of the specifics of Madeline's birth?" I ask.

"Definitely. For sure," she replies, unconvincingly.

"Madeline was born sixteen weeks prematurely," I continue, "and is in the NICU at the Grace Hospital. We are months away from a possible discharge, so I'm not sure this call is relevant right now."

"Right! Let's discuss your health then."

"I am well. I didn't have a difficult labour, so no tearing to recover from. I am getting sufficient rest and am eating well."

"Good to hear. Are you planning to breastfeed?"

"Yes. I've rented a pump through the hospital for now."

"Excellent. Researchers have found many benefits associated with breastfeeding, so you are giving your baby the best start possible. Do you have any questions? Any concerns about latching or production?"

"No." I sigh. "Madeline is nowhere near latching. They haven't even started feeding her and when they do, the dosage will be one cc. Milk production isn't my biggest concern at the moment."

The nurse latches on to my last statement. "And what is your biggest concern at the moment?" she asks.

I roll my eyes. Does this woman not understand what we're going through? Has she read my file?

"I am concerned for the health of my daughter," I say levelly.

"Of course. But since Madeline's birth, have you been able to laugh and see the funny side of things—as much as you always could, not quite so much now, definitely not so much now, or not at all?"

I'm silent. How do I word my answer? I haven't done much laughing lately. Who would? And I don't feel like quantifying my happiness, whether or not she has a form to fill out or not.

I take a deep breath. "Although I am seriously concerned about Madeline's health, I have a wonderful husband and mother. We are supported by many friends who are offering assistance however they can."

"So do you feel anxious or worried—for no good reason at all, hardly ever, sometimes, or not often?"

"I think I am in the best mental state I can be, all things considering."

The nurse is silent for a moment and I imagine I hear her click her pen off. "If you need any assistance in the days ahead," she says, "you will find my contact information in the blue folder you were given at discharge."

I say goodbye and end the call, then sink back into the pillows, wishing I could fade away.

Chapter 15

"AFTER YOU LEFT LAST NIGHT, MADELINE'S BREATHING WORSENED," says Nurse Bridget, with a strange look I've learned to recognize as "brace yourselves, things are about to get worse."

It's one day after my discharge, seventy-two hours after birth, and we're standing beside the incubator. Madeline looks much the same as she did at birth—crimson, fragile, a heartbreak in a box.

"Why the change?" Josh asks. "Is she tiring out like Dr. Fiala said she might?"

"Maybe," Bridget says. "This change is typical in a preemie after a few days of birth—she might need a rest—but it could also be a sign of infection. We'll talk on rounds, but the doctors will likely order more blood work."

Bridget looks serious—not worried, but definitely serious. She's Irish though. They're always pessimistic...or is that optimistic? I can't remember.

"What kind of infection could it be?" Josh asks.

"It could be anything. Hospitals are filthy places. We always wash our hands, but we are constantly pricking her and poking her. Something in the air could have entered during blood work. As a micro-preemie, she has zero immunity against anything floating around."

We peek at Madeline under the incubator blanket. She lies on her side, completely still except for the occasional flare or twitch of fingers. Her wee legs, angular sticks of tendons and bones, are separated by a rolled cloth. Her chest moves in and out as the ventilator forces air into her lungs, damaging tissue with every breath. She's connected to a tangle of lines—a mechanical ventilator hose into one of her miniscule nostrils, a feeding tube between her lips, three heart rate sensors and a carbon dioxide monitor stickered to her chest, an IV line held with globs of tape between her arm and a Styrofoam board, and an oxygen saturation sensor glowing red on her foot. The lines flow out of her incubator through a port sleeve, plugging into machines, feeding numbers on screens. Her well-being is revealed in those numbers, whether she's moving closer to us or slipping away.

Bridget opens the incubator doors. "I'm sorry," she says, flinging her dark red bangs out of her eyes with a toss of her head, "but you're going to see something nasty."

With one hand under Madeline's head and the other under her legs and bottom, Bridget flips Madeline onto her back. And, sure enough, Madeline's left arm is bloated and red, twice the size it should be.

"What happened?" I gasp.

"Last night, her IV line popped out of her vein, into her arm tissues. It should have been checked more frequently than it was, I'm afraid."

Bridget eyes me cautiously, perhaps seeing the fury billow inside of me. "I filed a patient report on the night nurse though," she goes on calmly. "It's all we can do right now. Madeline's veins are incredibly fragile. The damage could have happened very quickly."

I ease my forehead onto the top of the incubator as tears come. My poor darling Madeline! She's only a pound, a poor wrinkled pound of broken baby. I know accidents happen, but seriously, did the night nurse not check her IV at all? Madeline's having a horrible life without being neglected.

Josh rubs my neck and sighs. I know he's upset too and I should try to comfort him, but I can't manage it right now. I'm too consumed with my own anger.

Bridget offers me Kleenex. "I've given her pain medication. She's sleeping. She won't feel her arm."

"How can she not feel it?" I whisper. "I had an IV go bad when I was in hospital and it was incredibly painful! How can she not be suffering?"

Bridget bites her lip and changes tactics. "When she's grown and is having a wonderful life, she won't remember any of this. None of us remember being babies, no matter how much pain we were in. I am keeping a sharp eye on her IVs and I will certainly warn the next nurse. Okay?"

I meet Bridget's eyes and realize the pointlessness of my tears. They are only making things worse and, besides, the doctors are about to begin their daily rounds. I wipe my eyes and sit in a rocking chair near the incubator.

The medical team surrounds Madeline's incubator, Josh, and me in a large circle. The respiratory therapists, residents, neonatology fellows, dietician, and paediatric pharmacist gather with Dr. Fiala to assess Madeline. They all wear hospital-issued blue scrubs and sensible footwear—there's not a ridiculous pair of shoes between them—and introduce themselves in soft voices. Perhaps they're wary of us, afraid of hysterics, or perhaps they've seen Bridget's report on the night nurse and, noting the streaks of mascara on my cheeks, are treading carefully.

Aside from Dr. Fiala and Bridget, not one of them looks a day over thirty. But they all listen intently, scribbling down notes in thick binders, occasionally requesting clarification.

Bridget starts the assessment by reciting Madeline's vital statistics, and then a respiratory therapist summarizes Madeline's breathing—"Respiration is very shallow. We aren't getting much height to her breaths on the monitor and her oxygen saturation is very low. Her diaphragm is visibly retracting with each breath. We have increased her ventilation support so she can rest."

Dr. Fiala frowns. "Definitely, Madeline needs a rest," she says, "so why isn't the oxygen level on the ventilator higher? She has desaturated three or four times while I've been standing here in, what? Two minutes? If you are giving her a rest, give her a rest. Let her have the oxygen she needs."

As if on cue, Madeline's oxygen saturation alarm begins to ring. We all turn to watch the overhead monitor blink oxygen saturation percentages to our upturned, wincing faces.

88, 82, 74… all the way down to 53, sinks a number that should be in the 90's. 53, 48, 46. We hold our breaths, watching silently. Madeline's body is processing just whiffs of oxygen and the risk of neurological damage increases every time the number plummets.

"Turn up the oxygen," says Dr. Fiala.

The respiratory therapist twists the ventilator's oxygen dial and waits, but there's no effect, or at least not the one we want. The percentage sinks even lower: 42, 40, 39, 36, and Madeline's alarm goes into panic mode—higher, faster, louder. Although the machine refreshes, 36 percent blinks over and over again. Then, after half a dozen tense seconds, the number begins to recover: 47, 52, 66, 74, 79. We let out our breaths and shuffle our feet, but Dr. Fiala is not pleased.

"Madeline is on a ventilator!" she snaps. "Why this variability of oxygenation? This is the fourth time this has happened in ten minutes! We need blood work to check for infection and a chest x-ray as soon as possible. My guess is that her lungs are filling with fluid from an infection. Let's start her on a small dose of antibiotics to be on the safe side."

Residents scribble orders with scratchy pencils. One reaches for the ward telephone to call the x-ray technicians. Another fills out a laboratory form for blood work.

Dr. Fiala turns to us. "Mom, Dad—are you okay?"

I don't know how to answer. We're not okay. We're scared. But Josh nods and whispers, "Thank you for your time," so the doctor moves on. There's another baby, another struggling soul, a few feet away, complete with her own issues and heartbroken parents.

We remain by Madeline's incubator, stunned into silence, while Nurse Bridget prepares for blood work, laying needles and syringes in a straight line across a sterile countertop. "Go home, guys," she says softly, kindly. "Go home. There's nothing you can do here."

We inhale ragged breaths, stroke the incubator one more time, then trudge down the hall toward the elevators, wondering how we can possibly go on with the day.

• • •

"WHEN DOES YOUR MOM LEAVE?"

We're in the car. Josh is driving downtown to his office where I'll drop him off, then carry on home. We'll make this journey in reverse when we visit this evening. Until then, Josh will put on a smile and attend meetings like there is nothing going wrong in his life and I will hide at home with Mom. But she leaves soon, and Michael is only scheduled to teach for a few more days, so I'll have to start facing my students with the same bravery with which Josh faces his colleagues.

"Wednesday," I answer.

Josh nods. "Okay. Do we need to talk about anything?"

I shake my head. I don't want to talk. I want to crawl into a hole and stay there until Madeline no longer looks so awful.

"Are you sure you're okay?" Josh presses.

"You can't wave a magic wand and make me okay. No one can."

Josh pulls into a "no parking" zone and gets out of the car. I slide across the front seat, behind the steering wheel.

"Don't worry about me," I say, forcing a smile.

He shrugs, then kisses my cheek and slams the door shut.

Chapter 16

I STILL FEEL PREGNANT. MADELINE WAS SUPPOSED TO COME IN July and it's only March.

I am at Fabricland, getting supplies so Mom can sew softer linens than the hospital-issued ones for Madeline's incubator. I idle the car, debating whether to park in an expectant mother spot or in a lonely spot at the far end of the parking lot. I've gotten used to parking in the spaces marked with a pink silhouette of a heavily pregnant woman. The figure has a ponytail and a bigger stomach than Bobbi McCaughey had when she was pregnant with septuplets. You can't miss those signs. But I realize I no longer qualify for this perk. I am nothing, not expectant and hardly a mother.

Silly as it may be, I pull into the expectant mother parking spot anyway. Pretending is pointless, but it seems unfair that I've had a baby but can't be happy about it.

I step inside the fabric store and am overwhelmed. Overhead music screeches. Buttons, needles, hooks and eyes all bounce off the shelves in weird optical illusions. Colourful bolts of spring fabric compete for my attention. Somehow, I find the Velcro dots, yards of flannel, and soft pink thread that Mom needs, then line up at the cash register.

But just as I'm second in line to the till, a wiry woman dashes in front of me, turning briefly to twitter some inane thing at me. Under normal circumstances, her rudeness would have annoyed me and I might have stared back with raised eyebrows and an incredulous look. But today I feel a surge of panic. I want to curl up on the floor and cry, or grab the woman's bony shoulders and shake her until her stupid head rattles.

"How dare you jump the line!" I want to yell. "You are a nasty, rude, horrible person! Do you know what my life is like? Do you know how scared I am?"

But I swallow back my unreasonableness and blink away my tears. I shouldn't be out in public. I should be in bed with the blinds pulled. But hibernating isn't an option.

"This too shall pass," I whisper to myself. "Find your new normal, Amy."

But what is normal when Madeline lies in an incubator, fighting for her life? What is normal when ventilator stickers gouge her cheeks and her fragile skin weeps and bleeds? I refuse to accept this as normal. I want Madeline to either improve or go to sleep forever, and there is nothing normal about that. Perhaps if I knew what was going to happen, I could wrap my head around it, but I don't know what to mourn.

I eventually pay for my items, then escape the store. Warmer temperatures have arrived, so the parking lot is wet with runoff from melting snow. The latest, freshest layers of snow are gone now and old, gravel-grunged layers appear from below. Lost mittens emerge. Twiggy arms of disintegrated snowmen marinate in mud puddles. Spring is here, but there is a whole lot of ugliness to deal with before summer will come.

• • •

"MADELINE MIGHT BE BETTER THIS EVENING," MOM SAYS HOPE-fully. "She'll have had the day to rest and maybe that's all she needed."

It's five o'clock and we're driving to the hospital. The linens Mom has sewn are in the back seat, neatly folded, stacked in a sealed plastic bag to keep them clean. A Tupperware container of sandwiches for Josh sits on the console between Mom and me.

"Maybe so," I say, changing lanes to avoid a slow driver. I notice Mom's right foot press an imaginary brake. "Sorry," I mutter.

"You need to be more patient, Amy. If the speed limit is a hundred, that's what you should be doing."

"Yep." I ease down to a hundred and ten. The road is dry and clear of traffic. A bit of hustle is hardly endangering our lives; besides, a heavy foot is a by-product of an efficient nature. Why should I waste time sitting behind a nervous driver?

But Mom isn't finished. "Madeline needs a mother, you know. If you die on the Queensway, will that help anything?"

"You're right."

I turn on CBC Radio One's *All in a Day* for a distraction. The topic is the Senate spending scandal and frequent promos for the evening news only refer to the carnage in Syria. The show isn't doing its stated purpose of helping me "unwind after a hectic day," so I shut it off.

"Your dad is prepping the air seeder for wheat." Mom reads a text on her phone. "We may do some flax this year too. It's best to let a year or two go between canola. You have to let the land recover."

"Yep." I sigh irritably. My parents assume I forgot everything I ever knew the second I left the farm, including the principles of crop rotation.

"Did I tell you we've ordered chicks?" Mom asks. "Seventy-five of them. We'll keep them for laying hens. Maybe we'll get some geese too though I've never cooked goose before. I'll have to research it on the internet."

"You mean Google it."

"Since when did Google become a verb?"

"It is, Mom."

"Well, anyway, Cece and Marek will love the chicks, but I expect Kara and Serena will be frightened."

Mom speaks warmly of her grandchildren, my sister's kids. I can picture them with cheeky grins and dirty faces, chattering away about baby chicks.

When I was a kid, I thought everyone who didn't live on a farm was miserable and I was sure I'd never leave. But by the time I was sixteen, the thought of never leaving prompted a tightness in my chest. There are a few forms of rural living and not all of them are pretty. Spending one's life gossiping over a sink of dirty dishes at the seniors' home, earning minimum wage, praying for the weekend is what happens to farm girls who skimp on education and don't marry sons of prosperous farmers. I knew enough not to risk it, so I did everything I could to get away, even if it only was to Brandon, Manitoba, population fifty thousand.

The Wheat City, as Brandon is called, was built on the banks of the Assiniboine River, which winds its way across the prairies like cornelli lace across a sheet cake. A hash of box stores, train yards and a slaughterhouse, Brandon was also home to my alma mater, Brandon University. After finishing my first degree in music there, I completed a second at University of Alberta in Edmonton. It was then I renewed an earlier acquaintance with Josh. He was working for a cabinet minister in Ottawa and on work trips to Edmonton he'd look me up. After a winter of weekend visits and daily Skype calls, he proposed. Since he had a job and I had nothing but framed parchment, it made sense to start our marriage in Ottawa.

It may have been a long, multi-province journey from the farm to Ottawa but now, years later, I have no regrets. My life might not be glamorous, but at least it was the life I chose. It wasn't foisted upon me due to a lack of options.

But as we hurtle down the grey Queensway, corralled by concrete sound barriers, my childhood on the spacious farm seems blissfully uncomplicated.

I think of early spring mornings when I'd stomp through a thin layer of ice on water puddles on the way to feed the pet rabbits. Cool nights would have frozen whatever standing water had accumulated during the previous day's melting, and it was pure joy to crack through the ice. When temperatures warmed, my sisters and I would hunt down batches of baby kittens, combing through the canvas hay shelter, the dusty machine shed, or the tired granaries left empty by the previous generation of farmers. Often on a lead from Dad—"I saw Hisser heading into the fertilizer shed with a dead mouse"—we creep in, listening for piercing meows from the kittens. Sometimes we'd find them nursing, four or five tiny pusses all lined up, the mother-cat's tail flopping loudly to the dusty wood floor, a contented smirk on her face. We'd wait until they finished and then carry them up to the house to show Mom, the anxious mother-cat scampering along behind. It was all so uncomplicated.

My cellphone beeps a text message alert. I stealthily check it as Mom chimes, "Amy, it's illegal to text and drive. Let me do it for you."

She takes the phone and reads that Josh has taken a bus from work to a stop close to the hospital. He's walking towards the hospital now.

We're still ten minutes away, stuck in traffic as the last clog of rush hour forms between the downtown and the off-ramp I take. We creep along, bumper to bumper, which is just as well, as the pavement crumbles from thawing frost. Spring is a destructive force on Canadian roads; it can turn even the best-built road into an obstacle course.

I weave around the obvious potholes and tense against the unavoidable ridges tracing across the street. I turn east onto the hospital's street, which is only in slightly better shape, and spot Josh ahead on the sidewalk, nearly at the hospital. I pull into a driveway ahead of him and wait for him to catch up. He looks worn out as he chucks his work bag across the back seat and slams the door behind him.

"Hey," I say.

"Hey."

"How are you?"

"Tired."

"Me too."

Mom hands him a sandwich.

"No word from the hospital on your cell?" I ask.

"No."

Nearly monosyllabic conversation is becoming increasingly typical for us. Too tired to talk, we usually don't bother.

I pull onto the hospital campus and up the ramp to the parking garage. A spot is open on the main floor, though a silver BMW is ineptly parked beside it, one tire straddling the faded yellow line.

"It's too tight, Amy," Josh warns as I manoeuvre the car into a sharp turn.

"It's fine," I say and squeak, inch by inch, into the parking space. In the rear-view mirror, I see Josh roll his eyes.

"Go out the left side, Josh," I snap. "Can you get out, Mom?"

"I'm fine."

We all slide out carefully, avoiding contact with the salt-covered cars. It's a bad time of year to keep vehicles clean in Ottawa. The city spreads truckloads of salt every time the temperature dips below freezing, which in March is nearly every day. The muddy brine encrusts vehicles, rusting them out. It's an automotive cancer contracted simply by driving.

Munching on the sandwich, Josh leads us down the dimly lit parkade staircase. We walk in mincing steps on the gravel scattered over the concrete. At the bottom of the stairs, Josh shoves the heavy door open against the wind.

It always seems blustery at the entrance to the parking garage. Big gusts funnel between the hospital and the garage, swirling up dust and gravel. The wind isn't warm yet either. It's sharp and cold, and stings the cheeks.

At the main entrance, we hold the door for an elderly man. He clutches a small bundle of carnations in one hand and a Tim Hortons sack in the other. He's weather-beaten and hunched, likely a reduction of his former self. I wonder if he's visiting his wife in one of the depressing wards like Geriatric Oncology or Cardiovascular Intensive Care.

We take the elevator up to the eighth floor and wind our way through the hallways. At the NICU, a pink cardboard heart is taped to the door. Pastel foam stickers spell out "NICU" in a simple arch. We brush past the heart, into a small waiting room outfitted with a large metal sink, a few coat hooks, and some ratty furniture. The ward clerk peers out from behind the glass window and asks us to wait. Madeline's room is too busy for visitors, she says. This is often the case when we visit. If a resuscitation is in progress or if a baby is in the middle of a procedure, then parents aren't allowed in.

We sit down, three adults spread over two threadbare armchairs and a child-size stool at a table loaded with colouring books. There are a few magazines, outdated and donated, but we all look at our cellphones anyway.

I have a screenful of unread emails from family and friends, all replies to a picture I sent yesterday. In the picture, I'm cupping Madeline's legs in my hand for size perspective. The severity of Madeline's prematurity is obvious, and replies to the email are filled with shock and sadness—"I can't stop crying when I look at these" or "I'm sure she's a fighter. I'm sure."

I punch out responses as I wait. A text here. A two-line email there. Something to let our loved ones know we appreciate their concern.

We all glance up as the hallway door opens. Two kids walk in and peer about nervously. No more than seventeen years old themselves, the girl and boy are uncared-for creatures. They look scraggly and malnourished, a bit dead in the eyes.

The girl's too-black dyed hair falls flat over her thin shoulders and her bloated, post-birth stomach hangs over the waistband of skinny jeans. Her bowed legs, jammed into massive winter boots, attach to her body at peculiar angles. She sucks back the last few drops of a thirty-two-ounce soda through a straw, tosses the cup into the garbage. She washes her hands while the boy—likely her baby's father, God help that child—slumps against the wall, his shiny, shoulder-length hair hanging flat against his pimply face. Rings, plugs, sticks, and stones protrude through his lips and ears. The boy is scrawny, but his pants haven't been informed. They're three sizes too big, sinking and sagging every direction.

The clerk calls out to him, "Wash your hands, please."

He ignores her and heads toward the door to the ward. Josh steps in front of the couple, his arms folded.

"Go wash your hands," Josh levels.

"I just did, man, like, before," the boy mumbles without eye contact.

"Now," Josh says calmly.

The boy sniffs dismissively and steps around Josh. Suddenly I find myself between the boy and the door, pointing dramatically toward the sink.

"You!" I snap, my adrenaline throbbing. "Right now. Wash!"

The boy hops back to the sink for a minimal attempt at filth removal, then scuttles past us. For the second time in one evening, Josh rolls his eyes. I decide it's a reaction to the boy, not to me, and I sink back into a chair in time to see Mom smile and shake her head, just a little.

I don't especially care if either Mom or Josh think I've overreacted. Germs in the NICU are deadly. Hand-washing is the least one can do to avoid the spread of infectious diseases.

On the other side of the clerk's glass wall, Phyllis, the head nurse in the NICU, punches a number into an old, boxy-looking telephone. She leans back in a swivel chair like an aging police officer after a night on the beat and takes swigs of coffee. After a quick exchange of pleasantries, Phyllis begins to discuss a mother, likely the one who just came through the waiting room.

"Well, she's a super-loser," Phyllis says into the receiver, "but shockingly enough that baby tested clean. Well, a bit of Prozac, but no crack. I know; I was surprised too. Children's Aid Society will be with her 24/7 until those papers get signed. Yeah, we're babysitting until they can arrange a home. God love that social worker, Connie—do you know her? Yeah, yeah. That's her. Patient as anything, and the boyfriend is a real doozy too. I'd have punched him by now myself."

Nearing retirement, Phyllis has likely seen everything over a long career in public health. She hangs up the phone a minute later and goes to check on Madeline's room. When she returns, she looks hesitant.

"Just parents tonight. No grandma," she says. "Madeline is not at her best. Your nurse will explain, but we've had her bowels x-rayed. It's possible that they're infected. You can go in now."

Josh and I hold hands and walk into Room A, the room with the weakest, most ill babies. At Madeline's incubator, Nurse Bridget stands with her arms folded. She looks puzzled.

"Madeline's not having a good day today," she says, "and we're not sure why."

Madeline lies very still under a blue jaundice lamp that makes her skin the colour of grape-flavoured Bubbilicious chewing gum. She doesn't wave her limbs or move her head, she just lies still, covered in wires. The ventilator tube has been moved from her mouth to her nose so the cracks in her thin, purple lips are visible.

"What's going on?" Josh asks.

"We don't know. An infection is likely but the lab results are coming clean."

"Which means?"

"Maybe she has something other than an infection. Maybe the loss of blood from her heart murmur is exhausting her. Maybe the bug is taking a long time to grow in the lab—some bugs do, which is unfortunate because we can't treat something specifically until we know what it is. For now, we're using a 'catch-all' antibiotic, to be safe."

"What about the bowel x-ray?" I ask. "Phyllis mentioned it."

"It's an exploratory measure. There's a possibility of necrotizing enterocolitis, or NEC, which is basically ill health in the bowel. Depending on the severity, it could cause inflammation, perforation, or tissue death. All of her tissues are incredibly fragile. Also, her diaper rash got away on us. We can't change her diaper very often because it upsets her, so unfortunately her little bottom is bleeding right through the diaper cream."

"Oh, Bridget," I groan. "Is she in pain?"

"Most likely," Bridget says softly. "That's why she's so still tonight. We have her on fentanyl, a sedative. Unfortunately, its major side effect is decreased respiration so, of course, we can't leave her on that for too long. We'll have the x-ray results back by tomorrow, so try not to worry between now and then about her bowel. We're coping with everything else."

Bridget returns to her charting, her efforts lit by a glowing desk lamp, and Josh and I pull chairs to the side of the incubator. From these high stools, we watch Madeline sleep and try not to worry, but that's impossible. How can we "not worry," as if worry is a switch that can be flicked on or off? There's no off-switch to worry for parents of sick children.

We sit as close to Madeline as we can get, but still I want to be closer. I want to pick Madeline up and rock her against my chest.

I want her to know how much I love her. But she sleeps in another world, oblivious to the chaos around her.

Monitors beep and alarms rings. More often than not, Madeline's oxygen saturation level dips, sometimes making a quick return and other times sinking lower and lower until Bridget increases the amount of oxygen that streams through the ventilator line. The constant call of the alarms unnerves me. The nurses say they hear the alarms in their dreams and I believe them. The ringing is relentless. If Madeline's oxygen level doesn't dip, her neighbour's or the baby's around the corner does. These poor little ones are all on mechanical ventilators, for pity's sake, but they still can't get enough oxygen.

Josh puts his arm around me. "She'll come along," he whispers. "It's going to take time."

"But what about this infection, Josh? If they can't find it, she's going to get worse."

"We don't know she has an infection."

"What then? Her oxygenation is all over the place, and she's on a ventilator!"

He kisses my forehead and we fall silent. Madeline lies on one side of thick plastic walls; we, on the other. We can't help her. We can only watch and dream of better days.

Perhaps other parents picture their children riding bikes or winning spelling bees. We dream of Madeline breathing on her own, without any machine to help her. How beautiful it would be to watch her breathe a breath, a magnificent intake of air into capacious lungs, a feat only matched by an exhale of equal enthusiasm. Maybe then, after completing the very act of survival, she might do it again. And again. And again. And maybe she would do it for the rest of her life. It's such a beautiful dream, so simple yet so complex. And it feels so far away.

After a half hour of careful watching, we leave the side of the incubator. There's really nothing we can do to be helpful. We might as well go home and get some sleep.

In the hallway though, by the waiting room where Mom still reads magazines, the couple from earlier hug each other. The girl sobs and the boy does his best to comfort her. "She's so little!" I hear the girl weep. "What will happen to my baby?"

Chapter 17

IT'S WEDNESDAY MORNING, A WEEK AFTER MADELINE'S BIRTH. She looks more fragile than the day she was born, if that's possible. Her mouth flops open in what looks like a constant gag from the tubes stuffed down her throat. Blood vessels spider their way across her bloated abdomen. Her skin seems even thinner, even more transparent. A new weeping sore appears every time a sticky sensor is moved and a nurse points out a dark spot under the skin of Madeline's tummy—it's her stomach, apparently.

I watch Madeline through stinging eyes. Just watching her makes me want to cry; my nerves are so frayed. I have just dropped off Mom at the airport and, though I've said many goodbyes at the airport, this goodbye was difficult. I will miss Mom, but I knew she couldn't stay forever. It was time for her to go home, time for me to manage without her.

I gave her a thank-you present at the airport, a picture of Madeline's wee face surrounded by the engraved line, "Thank you for helping, Grandma. Love, Madeline." It was sentimental gift, one that might be shuffled to the bottom of a drawer if Madeline doesn't survive, but Mom seemed touched. She put it in her purse, not her suitcase, as if she planned to look at it during the flight.

Hours later, I'm still blinking back tears as Dr. Fiala stands over the incubator, frowning through doctors' rounds. Josh had to attend a meeting at work, so I'm listening to the horribleness on my own.

"I'm so sorry," the doctor says, "but the x-ray showed that Madeline's bowels are severely inflamed. We have been holding her feeds for a couple of days and will continue to do so. We can't risk this getting worse. Also, I'm afraid there's no news from the lab about an infection, which is bad news in this case. Madeline has an infection somewhere, and every day we can't target it with specific antibiotics is a day lost."

I notice the doctor forces her eyes open to keep from crying, and then I realize she's mirroring me because, no matter how hard I stare, tears are coming. I can't stop them. Nurse Bridget hands me a box of Kleenex and I wipe at the streaks of mascara I know are forming on my cheeks. Unfortunately, Dr. Fiala isn't finished.

"We've taken a lot of blood for tests," she goes on, "so Madeline will soon need a transfusion. Part of our problem is that Madeline's heart is not efficient. Her last heart ultrasound showed that the murmur was large, but we can't treat it because the medication would interfere with the antibiotics. So we're caught. For now, we wait for lab results on the infection, hope that by holding feeds and treating the bowels with antibiotics the inflammation will decrease, and pray the heart murmur doesn't worsen. You have to understand, this is the most difficult time: when issues start piling up."

She bites her lip and I wonder how many hard cases she's lived through, how many unidentifiable ailments, heartbroken parents, and unpredictable conditions. Yes, this is her job, but I bet she wishes she were somewhere else. Somewhere warm. Somewhere far from all this misery.

"I'm not very happy right now," she says, exhaling.

Although obvious, her words are the most tragic thing she's said so far. They're a summary, a reminder of earlier counselling, of reality, of inevitability.

I stare back at her, my jaw trembling, my hands shaking. I wonder if everyone can hear my heart thumping, just above my left breast that's worn raw from the pumping machine. Do they see my panic? Do they watch me with careful eyes filled with sympathy or is it watchfulness? Do they wonder when I'm going to start wailing?

I don't want anyone to feel any worse than they already do, so I thank the team for their time, and they move on to the next baby.

Nurse Bridget takes my hand. "Are you okay?" she asks.

I shrug. My micro-preemie has an unidentifiable infection, an inflamed bowel, and a heart murmur that can't be treated. She's dropping weight and she only started at a pound plus a few ounces. In all honesty, I know the answer to Bridget's question: I'm not okay. Not at all. I'm a hair's breadth away from breaking down at any moment.

"I know this is hard for you," Bridget goes on, "and you want to be here as much as you can, but you need to make time to sleep and eat properly."

I nod. What she is saying is reasonable, just not very realistic. I wish I could press pause on my life so I could quietly sit and watch Madeline without bills and obligations mounting around me, but that isn't possible.

"When do you go back to work?" Bridget presses.

"Today. Josh is already back."

"And are you sleeping through the night?"

"No, I get up to pump. The lactation consultant said to do that for the first couple of weeks, to get a flow established."

Bridget shakes her head. "As of tomorrow, I'm off for ten days, but when I return I want you rested. Got it?"

"I just want to be still here in ten days," I say with defeat in my voice.

"Yeah, I know. I know."

There's no point in me staying, hovering over the incubator, waiting for changes that don't occur, panicking over those that do, but I feel guilty for walking away. With Madeline doing so poorly, the hours between morning and evening visits feel like a lifetime. She could be overcome by evening, gone forever, or she could be exactly as we left her in the morning, hooked up to a dozen machines, bobbing gently on some great sea that will carry her to one port or another.

I go home, as if my whole world isn't lying in a heated Plexiglas box, and make a bracing pot of coffee. I measure out the coffee grounds, spilling some, then flick the whole mess into the sink with a stale rag. I eat a sandwich, and then at one o'clock I practise a smile in the mirror. I dislike what I see—I'm pale. I'm tired looking—but it doesn't matter. My maternity leave is over. Whether or not I'm ready, it's time to go back to work.

. . .

"I WAS EXHAUSTED WHEN I HAD MY KIDS AND THEY WERE NORMAL births, so I've brought something for your supper." Beth unpacks a sturdy, fabric bag onto my hallway bench. She's a sympathetic adult student with a knack for cooking. "These burgers need a few minutes on the barbeque or on a pan. They are organic elk, actually, and should be served with the pickled zucchini slices and radicchio. There are some homemade brioche rolls as well and some watermelon and feta salad."

I'm overwhelmed. I am struggling to keep up with meals and the spread in front of me is ten times more brilliant than the slurry of chili currently bubbling in my crockpot,

"This is so amazing, Beth!" I exclaim. "I can't thank you enough."

"Don't mention it. I love cooking, and cooking for someone who needs it is so rewarding."

We walk down the hall, into my teaching studio. It's a small room, large enough for a glossy Heintzman upright and a sun-stained Howard grand to squeeze in front of garden doors. The grand piano is too loud for the size of the room, so I leave its lid down and let books grow on top of it in dusty stacks. I delude myself into believing that all the scores might be needed in a lesson but, in truth, the majority haven't been returned to the bookshelves that line the walls.

I sit on a hard chair beside the piano; Beth, on a squishy bench in front of the grand. She moves the bench in and out until her tall frame is comfortably accommodated.

"Okay!" she laughs. "I think I have finally mastered the F-sharp minor scale! Not that it's anything to really care about this week, eh?

"It's okay, Beth. Distraction is its own form of therapy," I say. "Harmonic form first. Two octaves. Hands together."

Beth tucks some loose wisps of her dark brown bob behind her ears, then plays the scale.

"Perfect, Beth." I say. "Let's hear your Chopin."

Beth launches into Chopin's "Waltz in A minor," a simple piece, well-loved by intermediate pianists though never published during Chopin's lifetime. He didn't think the melancholy sweetness was his best writing. Beth plays the waltz well, so well I catch myself thinking more about Madeline than about Chopin. But it's not fair to Beth, who is paying for intelligent advice, not vacant stares. I have to provide feedback. So by sheer willpower, I focus on what I see and hear.

I notice Beth hesitates on the downbeats. She probably knows the left-hand notes, but can't find them quickly enough to play them on time. Her keyboard geography is likely weak. Big jumps, hesitations before downbeats, quick glances to the hand—my diagnosis makes sense. I consider walking her through a harmonic analysis so she'd know what chords she was jumping to, but analysis isn't her strength, so the additional data might confuse her. Her pedalling could be clearer too. Perhaps listening for the low notes as chord fundamentals to be caught with the pedal would improve her awareness of those notes. More lilt on the downbeats would be good; she's far too heavy on beats two and three. I could recommend a little rubato. A bit of push and pull? More waltz-like?

The more I analyze, the more I assess, the more quickly time goes by. As Beth experiments with my suggestions, I write a practice assignment. By the end of her lesson, the images of alarms ringing and doctors frowning have faded. It's as if the hospital exists on another plane, in another life.

My next student is fourteen-year-old Carla. She eases the front door shut without a sound, bobbing her crimped blonde hair in my direction.

"Hello," she murmurs with a hesitant smile. "How's the baby?"

Carla seems nervous, as if her mother instructed her to be careful around me. I plaster on an amiable smile and pull a picture from my cluttered box of teaching supplies. It's the same picture I emailed to family and friends the other day. In it, I'm cradling Madeline's legs in my hand as lines, hoses, and wires weave all around. Madeline's legs are the same width as my middle fingers and her toes are barely formed.

Carla's eyes widen. "Oh, wow!" she gasps. "She's so tiny! Is she okay?"

I swallow hard. I cannot cry in front of a student. I cannot.

"She's not doing as well as she could," I say, "but we have every hope that she will improve."

My answer is based in self-preservation, motivation by denial. If I pretend everything is a moment away from improving, then maybe it actually will.

Seemingly satisfied with my answer, Carla begins by playing her technique assignment. I determine to care about missed F-sharps, confused scale fingering, and unsteady rhythm, but my resolve quickly slips. I get antsy. I ask Carla for another rendering of a particularly troublesome scale, then stealthily check my phone. There's a text from Josh: "Please call me when you get the chance. The hospital called. We need to talk."

I am three minutes into Carla's lesson with forty-two more minutes to go, but I won't wait to call Josh.

"Carla, would you write out the fingering for the E-flat major scale?" I ask. "You can use my technique book as a guide. I need a second."

Carla nods and I step into the entrance hallway, shutting the studio door behind me. The tiled floor feels icy under my feet, so I sit on the carpeted stairs and call Josh.

"What's wrong?" I ask when he answers.

"The hospital needs our permission to do a spinal tap."

"Why a spinal tap?"

"They are trying to determine if Madeline has a brain infection because they can't find an infection in any of the blood work and she keeps getting sicker."

"Shoot."

"Yeah. It's an exploratory measure, though, and is fairly simple. They use a needle to collect fluid from her spine."

"If there was a brain infection, could they do anything about it?"

"I imagine so, but we're not at that stage yet."

"No, I know. Did you give permission?"

"Yes. I assumed that you would agree if it's recommended."

"Yes, of course. Keep me posted. I have to go."

I beep off the phone and return to the lesson. Carla has written out the right-hand fingering for an E-flat major scale without consulting the guide I left her.

"Okay, Carla." I speak slowly to neutralize the harried frustration in my voice. "If E-flat major has three flats, and it does, then the first note of the scale is a black note. Would you start with a thumb?"

"Maybe I should look at your technique guide for a second." Carla opens the book, flips past the index, and eventually locates E-flat major by randomly turning the pages back and forth. She writes out the scale fingering so slowly I want to snap, "Oh, speed up, for crying out loud!" but I swallow hard and envision what is happening in the NICU.

Madeline will be positioned in the fetal position so her vertebrae will be as exposed as possible. Antiseptic and anesthetic will be applied, then a needle will be eased into Madeline's back by a hand most steady, through layers of skin and muscle, right into the spine. Pull! There'll be a miniscule whoosh of fluid—a tiny bit will do—then the needle will be pulled out. Mission accomplished. I hate to think of it, yet I do, staring into space over the top of the piano, floating away. After a minute, I realize with a jolt that Carla has finished writing out the fingering and is staring at me, wide-eyed.

"Oh...good, great, Carla," I stammer, dragging myself back to the lesson like a swimmer climbing out of a pool, forces weighing down the body. "Well done. I'll hear that scale next week. Could we start with the Mozart minuet?"

Carla nods, then begins. But soon her errant right-hand pinky finger strikes a wrong note, and then another. I want to reach over and play the minuet myself for the sake of Mozart's nerves if not my own, but Carla sets her jaw, squints at the music and begins again, a little more slowly, at my recommendation.

I sigh on the inside—this is going to be a very long day.

• • •

HOURS LATER, JOSH ARRIVES HOME. HE DASHES UPSTAIRS TO CHANGE out of his suit as I trail after him, blowing on a bowl of hot chili. I'm on a short supper break and am desperate to talk, even for a few minutes.

"Did the hospital say when they'd have the spinal tap results?" I ask.

"Not sure. Fairly quickly I think."

Josh lays his pants and jacket over the back of a chair and unbuttons his absurdly creased collared shirt. Undoubtedly, it came from the closet that creased. I hope he didn't take his jacket off at work. As a Parliamentary Assistant in the House of Commons, Josh could in theory run into the Prime Minister in the course of a day. It would be unfortunate to encounter one of the leaders of the Free World sporting a shirt that looks slept in.

"Did they say how Madeline was this afternoon?" I ask.

"The same. They gave her a transfusion. It will delay her own red blood cell growth, but something had to be done. She was getting drawn down."

Josh pulls on a grey sweater over his blue jeans. The sweater looks big and the belt is hooked on a new, tighter notch. He's lost weight; I'm sure of it.

"Josh, are you eating?"

"Of course."

"What did you have for lunch?"

"I couldn't find leftovers in the fridge and I didn't want to waste money at the cafeteria so I grabbed an apple."

"That's what I thought. Sorry—I've gotten behind with cooking. There's chilli in the crockpot for tonight though. Get some before you go to the hospital. Beth brought food, so that will be tomorrow night's dinner."

Josh thumps down to the kitchen, shoulders down. I need to breast pump so Josh can take some milk to the hospital. If they restart Madeline's feeds, I want her to have fresh milk.

I pull my top over my head and sit in front of the breast pump, a frightening-looking device of medieval magnitude plopped on an ottoman. It operates by suction, rather like a pulsating vacuum. Narrow plastic tubing connects from the machine at one end to shields at the other. Milk drops into bottles through valves.

I can surf the internet while pumping if I use my knees to balance my laptop. If managed correctly, the laptop braces the shields against me, leaving at least one of my hands free for typing. It's a delicate arrangement, which usually results in something slipping, and warm sticky milk spilling all over me, but tonight I manage without mishap.

I browse through the depressing news headlines: "Syrian government guerrilla fighters sent to Iran for training. Israeli Military Intelligence chief said that Syria is becoming a center of global jihad. UNICEF estimates hundreds of thousands of children are displaced." The reality is obvious: Syria is going to pieces and I can't imagine Madeline's birth would be much of a priority in the Syrian health care system at the moment.

After ten minutes of pumping, I've produced an inch of milk in both bottles. If Madeline's feeds are resumed, she'll only be given two cc's every four hours, so these bottles will last for quite a while.

I hear my first student of the evening let herself in, so I dress quickly, then pack the milk in a thermal bag with ice from the freezer. Josh stands in the kitchen over a sink full of dirty dishes, scarfing down a bowl of chilli. He reaches out, so I wrap my arms around him. He holds me for a few seconds, his hand at the back of my head, his lips on my forehead—a moment of peace in a day of panic. Then he mutters, "You seriously need to wash your hair, Babe."

"Yeah, yeah, I know," I say, pushing his arms away. "It's practically crawling."

I run downstairs to the teaching studio and greet my student. I have three more hours of cautious looks, hesitant fingers, and jangled nerves, and I really don't want to deal with lost notebooks and ignored fingering. I don't want to teach with the nasty thought in the back of my mind: what if Madeline doesn't make it? Will I be able to face another teaching year, another round of kids?

As morbid as my thoughts are, they're the ones I want to think. They take less focus than the ones related to teaching.

• • •

"WHAT IS IT?" I ASK HOPEFULLY. "IS SHE BETTER?"

It's ten o'clock that night, and Josh has returned from the hospital, looking inexplicably happy.

"She's no worse. But it was time to change the incubator, so I got to hold her."

"How did she handle it?"

"Not too badly. It was a quick transfer, thirty seconds at most, and she was still hooked up to her ventilator, so there wasn't much opportunity for her to get upset. It was scary though. She felt like nothing, just a pound and a bit. So light."

Josh hands me the camera. "Nurse Bridget took a couple of pictures for you."

I sit down on the steps to click through the camera's image review. In Josh's arms, Madeline is barely noticeable. She's wrapped in blankets, tucked close to his blue-robed chest to protect against chills. Josh's smile is tentative, pleased, but worried too.

"Was it exciting to hold her?" I ask as he sits down beside me.

"I suppose. It was nerve-wracking though. She's my daughter, but I felt I was breaking rules by touching her."

"I'm sorry I wasn't there. I feel like a bad mother."

"It's okay."

Josh lays his head on my shoulder and I press it into my neck. Josh's face is always gentle, but when he talked about holding Madeline tonight there was a glow about it too. It's not easy to talk about your child clutching at life in an incubator. Your eyes smart and your throat thickens. A lot of swallowing is needed, and even if your mouth smiles your eyes stay sad.

We're still on the stairs a minute later, almost dozing, when the telephone rings. The telephone ringing has taken on new significance since Madeline's birth. We always assume it's the hospital calling with bad news.

Josh dashes up the stairs, pausing to check the caller ID. "It's the hospital," he says and I get a sinking feeling.

"Josh here," he answers, then walks into the kitchen, out of my earshot. It's better that way. He knows I don't want to hear him while he talks to a nurse. I read too much into the silences and sighs. Just give me the facts after the call.

Josh hangs up the phone, then climbs back down to the step I'm still sitting on. "They got the report from the lab," he says. "Madeline has an E. coli infection in her blood."

We stare at each other in disbelief. E. coli kills big people, never mind poor Madeline, only a week old and still just a pound.

A wave of vague impressions about E. coli from news headlines rolls through my mind. Beaches and lakes are put into lockdown over E. coli. Restaurants are closed. I can't think how Madeline would have contracted it. She wasn't swimming in Mooney's Bay or eating salad at Taco Bell.

"How did she get it?" I ask.

"Probably through a needle prick. Hospital air is dirty. They've already been in contact with the paediatric pharmacist, apparently. She suggested a totally different course of antibiotics than the one they've been using."

"So we've been wasting time with the other drugs." I sigh at the ceiling.

"They said Madeline is okay at the moment, not desaturating too much, but that it's going to be difficult in the next few days. Recovery could be slow."

We sit silently together, staring at the wall in front of us. The house is still, but my thoughts are racing.

"I'll text our parents the news," Josh says eventually, breaking the silence as he reaches for his cellphone on his hip.

"I'm going for a bath," I say, kissing his forehead, then trudging up the stairs. In the bathroom, I fill the tub, then sink into the hot water. I lie back against the ledge and close my eyes.

So much can happen in one day. We now know the mysterious ailment, but naming it only frightens me more. I feel guilty too. I should have been at the hospital tonight. I'm the mother. I should always be there. Teaching makes me feel so negligent, so absent.

Josh steps into the bathroom, shutting the door quickly to keep in the heat, then pulls himself on top of the counter. "Your mom has already responded to my text," he says. "She seems a bit panicked."

I snicker. Poor Mom. It really isn't funny though.

"She'll have her friends whipping out the prayers by midnight."

"And thank goodness," I say, loosening the elastic around my hair, then sinking low into the tub until only my face bobs above the water line.

"Indeed. We need all the prayers we can get."

I sit up suddenly, splashing a little. "I sometimes feel like I can't pray. It's too much work." I squeeze shampoo out of a nearly empty bottle, then rub it into my hair until it froths. "I keep praying, 'God save her. Don't let her die before she's even had a chance to live.'"

Josh sits on the floor and motions for me to turn around. He has a tumbler from beside the sink and he uses it to rinse out my hair, one careful cupful at a time.

"That's what friends are for," he says, his voice heavy with exhaustion. "The people that love you pray for you when you can't manage it."

I twist around to face him. His eyes are red and lined. Wrinkles trace his face. A few more whites sprout among the browns at his temples.

"Josh, you need to get some more rest. You look awful."

He nods half-heartedly, agreeing but acknowledging futility. There aren't enough hours in the day to visit the hospital twice, keep up with work, and stay rested.

"Grab a towel?" I ask.

Josh pulls a soft towel off a hook, and as I step onto the bath mat he wraps the towel around me and pulls me close, wet hair and all. "I love you, Babe," he whispers.

"I couldn't survive this without you," I say.

He kisses me, and my world regains a tiny bit of equilibrium.

Chapter 18

THE ENTIRE WARD IS READY FOR A LINE OF DOCTORS-IN-TRAINING to march out of the Physicians' Room behind a binder-laden neonatologist and start rounds. Nurses review case notes, carefully informing themselves of their babies' conditions. Respiratory therapists tinker with ventilators, adjusting knobs and oxygen lines, repositioning ventilator hoses. Elderly cleaning ladies smile and nod to compensate for their lack of English as they empty waste bins filled with packaging from needles and syringes, miniscule diapers, and rafts of paper towels from endless hand-washing routines. Ultrasound and x-ray technicians wheel massive machines around tight corners, announcing themselves in inquiring tones—"Head ultrasound, MacPherson?" or "Bowel x-ray, Walhinda?"

Josh and I perch on high, wheeled chairs at the incubator, waiting for doctors' rounds, as we do every morning. We want to know what will be the next step in Madeline's treatment, what calamity has befallen since yesterday. We wait with the rest of the ward, holding our breaths for whatever verdicts will be passed down today.

Paul, a stout young respiratory therapist from the "other side of the river"—Gatineau, Quebec—greets us cheerfully, his freckles disappearing into the folds of his broad grin. "Good news," he says, "I was able to turn down Madeline's ventilator PIP by a few points!"

"Wonderful, Paul," I say blankly, "but I can't remember what PIP stands for. Too many acronyms, I'm afraid."

"Of course." Paul bobs his head in deference to my ignorance. "PIP stands for 'peak inspiratory pressure,' basically the force we use to blow air into Madeline's lungs. If we use too little, the lungs won't get enough air and her oxygenation levels will drop. If we use too much, we damage lung tissue. When lungs are wet like Madeline's, a lot of pressure is required, so it's a good thing that she needs less PIP. Her lungs might be getting better."

"Maybe she's responding to the new antibiotics?"

"Perhaps. We'll know for sure if we're able to turn down her oxygen."

I lift the incubator blanket to peek at Madeline. She lies on her stomach, her tiny, sinuous legs tucked up against her bottom, her arms bent at ninety degrees beside her head. Her skin is foggy and mottled, not red like before.

Nurse Linda, a kindly woman with an odd juxtaposition of girlish freckles and matronly grey hair roots, opens the incubator doors, then changes her mind. She leans over the top of the incubator and whispers, "You know that carbon dioxide sensor that we have on Madeline? The little heated one?" We nod. "Well, I'm afraid it burned Madeline. It heats when it's first put on—the heat gives an accurate reading more quickly—but I'm not sure if it heated for too long or if burned in a short amount of time. Either way, you'll see a very bad sore on Madeline's side when I turn her."

Nurse Linda rotates Madeline and a quarter-sized, blood-caked scab appears, forming a constellation with sores from previous days. Although worse things might be happening below the surface of her skin, the wounds make the hair on the back of my neck stand on end. I feel Madeline's silent agony more acutely than if she were screaming, because even if she wanted to cry from pain she can't, not with a ventilator tube stuffed down her throat. Besides, she's too sick to protest.

My sister used to tell a story from her job at a nursing home: a patient with Alzheimer's disease would endlessly roam the halls crying, "I've got to get the cows in or Father will be so angry." Nothing the nurses would say could convinced her that the cows were in and she could rest. She was unreachable, lost in another world. Time had stopped for her.

Madeline is the opposite. Time hasn't even started for her. She's stuck in a world without thought. Alone in an incubator, waiting for time to pass, she's too sick to be touched, or spoken to. She doesn't know how much we love her. I'd like to think if she did, she'd be comforted. But when needles stab or sensors rip skin, her hands clench, her arms flail, and her respiration plummets. And there's not a single thing I can do. She suffers alone.

"Her skin will get thicker in time, Amy." Nurse Linda pats my shoulder. "She is responding to her new antibiotics, so that's good news! Maybe by the end of today, we can wean down her oxygen."

I know Linda is trying to make me feel better, but Madeline's broken and bleeding skin upsets me. I want to grab Linda by the shoulders and demand, "Is Madeline going to live or are we going to keep scuffing her up until the day she dies?" But there is no point. What can Linda tell me? She's no fortune teller.

"Why is Madeline so white and foggy-looking?" I ask.

"She's not producing red blood cells yet, and we are taking a lot of blood for tests," Linda says. "Basically, we're draining her and she's unable to replace what we're taking. We've already given her one transfusion, but we'll have to talk about another on rounds today."

"What does she weigh now?" Josh asks.

"She's taken a hit. It's normal for babies to lose ten percent of their birth weight in the first week, but I'm afraid Madeline is down from 630 grams to 520. That is a seventeen percent loss, which reflects how ill she's been."

Five hundred and twenty grams. Half a kilogram. A box of salt. A pound of butter.

Like a fragile bird shoved out of the nest too early, Madeline is a bundle of sick, underdeveloped organs held together by fragile bones, sourced with donated blood, covered in wounded, scarred skin. That she lives from one moment to the next seems miraculous to me.

Doctors' rounds begin at Madeline's incubator. Linda recites Madeline's vital statistics for the team and Paul joyfully recounts the two-point PIP reduction, though his announcement is undermined by the constant ringing of Madeline's oxygen saturation alarm. It seems Madeline's oxygen requirements are actually increasing, not decreasing, as he suggests.

"We may need to revisit the PIP levels, Paul," says Dr. Fiala. "I know the stronger the ventilator's air flow, the more damage to the lungs, but it's a vicious cycle: if we tire her out, then we'll be back where we started. I don't want her pushed too hard. Turn the ventilator back up."

Paul does what she asks with a defeated look. Everyone in the ward wants to see the patients improve, even if it's only by two points of PIP.

The doctor smiles a smile that has more sympathy than joy, but is a smile nonetheless. "Madeline has survived a week," she says, "and that's wonderful, but she has a lot of issues. We have her on powerful antibiotics for the E. coli—thank goodness the lab figured out what it was—and we'll continue holding the feeds until the bowel inflammation decreases. Soon we'll talk about treatment for the heart murmur. For now, she needs another blood transfusion. So long as nothing else goes wrong, we may make some progress. My time on-call here is done though," says Dr. Fiala. "You'll be seeing Dr. Lowry from now on."

"Thank so much for everything you've done," I say, reaching out to shake her hand.

The doctor grips my hand for a second, as if we can refer to the past week in a momentary hand-squeeze. Then, she moves on to another baby and another, for hours and hours, until twenty-odd babies have been seen.

At Madeline's incubator, Nurse Linda furiously pencils in the specifics of doctors' rounds onto Madeline's chart. Trends and tendencies, policies and priorities—the game of Madeline's life is played out on that chart. Miniscule grid boxes, each stuffed full of abbreviations, line up like chess squares, their fine-point figures contrasting only with the scrawl of nurses' signatures. In isolation, the bits of data might seem terrible, deadly even, but when viewed as a group, an entourage of statistics, they show Madeline is still alive. And if she can live for one week, then why not for two?

"Okay, here's the plan for the day," Nurse Linda says, stacking Madeline's chart against the order binder on the counter, "Madeline is scheduled for a head ultrasound later this morning to check for brain bleeds and a PICC line right away."

"What's a PICC line?" Josh asks.

"It's a tiny IV line that we feed through veins in the arm, up into the shoulder, until it reaches the superior vena cava. The SVC, as we call it, flows right into the heart. The line can stay in for a week or two and can be used to give medications. An IV line is eliminated—they tend to be problematic, as you know—and Madeline will experience less pain in the long run. We can check the line's position by ultrasound. It's a tricky procedure, but no more traumatic for her than an IV insertion. All the same equipment is used."

Linda gestures to needles, catheters, gauze, towels, tape all lined up across the sterilized counter like assembly-line parts. Ordered. Organized. Ready for action.

"And don't worry," she says. "We'll give her sucrose to help with the pain."

As much as I hate needles, I would have taken any number of stabs from a shaky-handed student nurse than have Madeline needled one more time, even by an experienced nurse. But that isn't an option. It has to be Madeline that suffers.

We whisper goodbyes to Madeline, then trudge to the car. It's only mid-morning, but we're already exhausted.

• • •

"COLONEL BY OR THE QUEENSWAY?" I ASK, SLIPPING BEHIND THE steering wheel. Josh has an eleven o'clock meeting to be dropped off for.

"Queensway."

Our journey is mostly south to north to Parliament Hill, the noble cliff overlooking the Ottawa River, but I humour Josh and backtrack to the east-west Queensway for one minute of highway speed before returning to the slower side streets.

We approach the downtown alongside the historic Rideau Canal, past the University of Ottawa. The turning lanes slow to a crawl as students fill the sidewalks, dashing from one class to another. They annoy me and my annoyance surprises me. It's not been long since I was one of them, but I feel the chasms between us. They all look weird to me—geek chic glasses, Peter Pan collars, fedoras on girls, fuchsia skinny jeans on boys. I don't understand them, nor do I want to.

After a left turn, away from the campus, I'm stopped at the crosswalk light in front of City Hall. The crosswalk is oddly placed—streets don't intersect—so it must have been built to allow City Hall staff to cross to Confederation Park without having to walk the half-block to the nearest set of lights. We watch several bureaucrats saunter by—desk-bloated stomachs, ID tags bouncing around necks, coffees and brown pastry bags in hand. Even they seem more carefree than us.

Further up the street, I pull over in front of a loading dock, under a sign that reads, "Do not even think of parking here." Josh hops out and calls goodbye, his workbag bouncing on his hip.

It's only 10:47 AM and I don't teach until 12:30, so I begin a plan, a self-indulgent, sugary plan. Since Madeline's birth, I have been out of my mind for sweets. Maybe it's the stress, or maybe my body needs a few extra calories for milk production. Either way, my need for sugar almost feels like a medical condition. The Flour Shoppe, a luxurious cupcakery, is only a few blocks away. I can swing by and still have time to pick up groceries before teaching. I pull back into traffic, and head south toward the Shoppe.

It has been said that downtown Ottawa can be split in two distinct districts. North of Laurier, the House of Commons and its subsidiary buildings scatter over Parliament Hill, Wellington and Sparks Streets. The Supreme Court and Libraries and Archives stand to the west; the National War Memorial, Chateau Laurier, and the Convention Centre, slightly to the east. Filling the blocks between these noble edifices are high commissions and embassies, lawyers and lobbyists, public relation experts and bureaucratic beehives. South of Laurier though, the city changes. Independent coffee shops replace Starbucks. Accountants and dentists outnumber industry associations and image consultants. Speciality shops sell comic books and art supplies instead of newspapers. And, fortunately for me, a charming shop sells sugar to addicts.

I find a spot in front of the shop that requires little from my limited parallel-parking skills, and as I get out of the car I smell whiffs of sugar floating in the air.

The Flour Shoppe is done up as a modern Parisian patisserie. White cupboards and panelling contrast with a royal purple ceiling. Ornately framed chalkboards list daily specials under the glow of pot lights. Ostentatious chandeliers sparkle over spindled cake covers. In the display case, row after row of perfectly formed cupcakes line up, their buttercream icing swirling in flawless swishes, left to right, each rotation growing more heavenward with identical inclination. Tiny pinpricks of popped air bubbles imply the icing was whipped into a frenzy before it was delicately applied to the tops of the rich, crumbly cupcakes.

I select two Earl Grey with lemon buttercream, two mocha with espresso, and two maple cream cupcakes. The shop assistant gingerly lifts each cupcake into a box, then ties it all up with a ribbon the shade of violets in the sunshine.

As I turn to leave, a wee girl, maybe four years old, catches my eye. Her eyes are bright; her lips, the shade of strawberries. Spiral curls in pigtails frame her little face. She presses her nose to the glass display window and squeaks, "I can't decide! Mommy, can I have two?"

Her mother smiles and says, "Just one," to which the little girl scrunches up her face, deep in thought.

She's so beautiful. So perfect. Her skin is thick and healthy, not red and ragged and raw. Her eyes sparkle and she's quite articulate for one so little. She seems blessed with a clever brain in a pretty head, and she's living a moment I want for Madeline. To be with your mother in a magical cupcake shop—could there be a better moment in childhood?

My eyes fill with tears, so I hurry to the car and slam the door shut behind me. I have to get away from that little girl. She's making me too sad. Far too sad.

I untie the cupcake box and choose an earl grey cupcake for starters. Head back, cake in—I savour the flavour, one tiny bit at a time, revelling in the escape from my own little girl and the painfully beautiful one in the shop.

I think of birthday cakes from my childhood, the delicious ones that Mom made with real butter and sugar, not the oily ones bought fully decorated at the bakery shelf now, chock full of artificial substitutes. My fourth birthday cake sticks out in my memory for some reason. It was a chocolate cake with Smarties arranged to look like a balloon. Everyone sang to me while I sat on the kitchen island beside the cake. I was very proud of my four years and my cake.

But perhaps I don't remember the scene at all. When I think of it now, I see it from a high angle, probably the perspective of my dad's camera. Maybe I don't remember anything other than the picture in the album. Maybe it's all gone.

I brush crumbs from my fingers and point the car home to Kanata. I need to get groceries.

· · ·

"OH HELLO, AMY! HOW ARE YOU?"

I glance up, over a mound of navel oranges. A woman from the neighbourhood stands smiling, struggling to pick a flimsy plastic bag off a roll while keeping three Red Delicious apples from rolling out of her elbow.

"Hi—I'm okay, thanks."

"We've been thinking of dear Madeline! How is she?"

I rip off a few bananas and struggle with my own bag. "Well, due to her prematurity, she is breaking down under the strain of an E. coli infection and a heart murmur. Her bowel is inflamed and she's dropping weight. Her lungs are hardly functioning. She's not well, really. Things are quite touch and go."

My neighbour sighs, the apples forgotten for the moment. She places a well-manicured hand on my black wool coat sleeve and says, "My son was born four weeks premature, so I know exactly what you mean! I was so concerned, but I had an amazing nurse who sat me down and said that everything was going to be okay! And it was! You have to stay brave, because it will all work out." She emphasizes her words with hearty pats to my arm.

"Was your son unwell?" I ask, worried that I've missed something obvious. Was he born without functioning organs or massive brain damage?

"Jaundiced. Poor little guy! He had to stay under the lamp for a few days before we could bring him home. It broke my heart! He was so yellow, and I couldn't hold him while he was under the lamp. I remember sitting by his little incubator crying and crying. And now—you'd never know. No! He's out playing hockey and getting on so well with his saxophone. It's hard to believe he was premature. It will be the same for Madeline, you wait!"

I smile a half-hearted smile that doesn't quite make it up to my eyes and stuff the bananas into my bag. "I'm sorry, so nice to see you, but I've got to run."

"Of course! You must be so busy. I remember what it's like! Do keep us posted!"

I scurry away, wanting to scream in the middle of the grocery store—"Your kid wasn't premature, not at thirty-six weeks, and jaundice isn't a terminal condition! Hearing your story doesn't give me courage to face the day. How stupid can you be?"

But after a few minutes, while hyperventilating over the frozen meat bunker, I calm down. My neighbour was trying to make me feel better, and even though she probably wasn't even listening to what I was saying—too busy trying to remember the details of her son's jaundice—she was empathizing. Undoubtedly, I've said innumerable careless things myself. It's a human flaw.

I muddle through the rest of my shopping and drive home with a splitting headache—the back end of a cupcake-inspired sugar rush. I shouldn't have eaten all that cake on an empty stomach. At home, I stagger up the stairs to the kitchen and ease the groceries onto the floor.

On the kitchen counter, the answering machine blinks red. With trepidation, I press the play button, but it's only Josh: "Hey! Where are you? I've tried your cell, but it must still be on silent. NICU called. They got the PICC line in and the head ultrasound came back clear. No brain bleeds, thank goodness."

I sink into a kitchen chair and eat yet another cupcake, the velvety buttercream first, then the cake, sultry and subtle all at once. It will only make my head worse but I don't care. I just sit, sweating in my winter coat, bags of groceries around my feet, and enjoy the first bit of good news we've had in a while. Madeline—clear of brain bleeds. How marvellous. Now if only we can keep her alive to enjoy that beautiful brain of hers.

Chapter 19

JOSH AND I LIE AWAKE, WAITING FOR THE ALARM TO GO OFF.

"No calls from the hospital," I murmur. "I keep thinking about her in the night though. Poor monkey."

Josh drapes an arm over me and exhales into my neck. The room is filled with early morning light. It seems that spring is here; I hadn't noticed until now.

As if on cue, the phone rings, cutting through the stillness. I startle, then grab the receiver as "NICU" pops up on the call display.

"Hello! Amy speaking," I answer, a bit frantically.

"Hi—this is Phyllis from NICU. Your baby is okay, but I wanted to catch you early. Dr. Lowry would like to meet with you to discuss treatment options. Madeline's breathing worsened overnight."

"What happened?"

"Her oxygen saturation kept plummeting even though we increased her oxygen level. We also switched her to the jet ventilator. Paul will explain when you come in, but basically the jet has a constant air flow. We also ordered a chest x-ray."

"Are you thinking another infection?"

"Definitely. The difficulties seem to be centring in the lungs this time, so perhaps it's pneumonia."

Phyllis sounds exhausted despite the fact it's only 6:58 AM. Maybe that's what happens to you after you've told parents that their child, despite being on a ventilator, isn't getting enough air and is getting worse by the hour.

I hang up the phone, then crawl across the bed to wrap my arms around Josh. He sits hunched, his back to me, legs over the side of the bed, waiting to hear what was so important that the head nurse would call at the crack of dawn.

"Madeline's oxygen requirements increased last night, so they switched her to a more supportive ventilator. They're going to do an x-ray and Dr. Lowry wants to discuss treatment options."

"Did she say what kind of treatment?"

"No, just that it's probably a new bug."

"We knew this could happen."

"I had hoped Madeline would have longer to recover between infections. Some time for her to build reserves after the E. coli."

I flop back onto the pillow and pull the covers over my head. The day is too depressing to face.

BEEP-A-BEEP-A-BEEP! Josh's phone alarm blasts. He swats at it, inadvertently knocking it onto the floor, under the bed. He grunts with exertion as he picks it up. "I'm going to make coffee," he mutters, shutting off his phone, then shuffling toward the stairs.

I close my eyes and wish I could escape. But even if I huddle under blankets all day, gloom will still perch on the end of the bed like a waiting vulture. I've nothing to gain by tucking up in a ball and crying. Despair will swoop, and what comes after that? I don't want to think.

I fling back the covers and pad down the hall to bathroom. In the corner of the mirror, I've tucked my bravery card, my inspiration for getting out of bed in the morning. It's just a 3″ × 5″ filing card, but on it I've scribbled anything that makes me feel remotely better:

Keep on believing.
God can do anything.
Where there's life, there's hope.
Maybe the next visit will be better.

I chant my mantras as I squint into the mirror. My hair needs a serious touch-up. The mousy brown roots are winning a war over the blonde. My eyebrows need thinning. My face looks sallow without makeup. I slide my contacts in—left eye first, then the right—and confirm my previous appraisal: work is definitely needed.

I can't fix the dark roots, but I part my hair at a different angle and mask them slightly. I tweeze the strays that edge my eyebrows, creating some order from the chaos. I wait a full minute for hot water to bubble up the pipes to the third-floor bathroom before soaking a facecloth. I scrub my neck and shoulders. Some of their tension dissipates as the heat penetrates, but still I'm tense. Every part of me feels clenched together by sheer willpower. I want it all to release, but it won't. Not yet.

Josh opens the bathroom door wide enough to slide a mug of steaming coffee onto the counter.

"Ta," I say, lifting the thick clay mug under my nose to breathe in the fragrance. It's a strong Starbucks dark roast, enough to wake you up with the smell alone. I take one sip, then another, enjoying the warmth spreading down to my belly.

I pull my over-stuffed makeup bag from a shelf above the toilet and consider its contents: creams, powders, pencils, brushes.

I've always worn makeup, from sixteen on, perhaps a little too much, perhaps a little garishly. It used to drive my mother mad. "You have beautiful young skin," she'd complain. "Why cover it?" But I don't use makeup today to look older or more sophisticated. I use it so I don't look like I'm falling apart. No one ever suspects a well-turned out mother wearing diamond earrings and lipstick to be on the edge, do they? It's the mother with scraggly hair and dull eyes, the one wearing sweat pants—she's the one suspected of losing her grip on reality. And anyway, I don't buy into the "natural is best" attitude. Preaching the evils of makeup is just a marketing ploy by soap companies. Give us women a break. We have enough to deal with without feeling guilty over wearing mascara.

I work from the top of my makeup bag to the bottom. By the time I'm finished, I look slightly less haggard than I feel, which I consider a success. I sip more coffee, then return to the bedroom to survey my closet.

Nothing jumps out at me as the thing to wear. Visiting your infant in the NICU—that's not really a tableau in the Sears catalogue, is it?

I settle on a steel-grey pencil dress with a thin aqua sweater, then dress quickly, one eye on the clock. Queensway traffic can be frustratingly slow early in the morning, and I don't want us to be late for rounds. I practise a smile in the mirror. A few new wrinkles appear around my eyes. I try another smile, one with less upward pull on the cheeks and scrunching around the eyes, but the wrinkles are still there.

"I can do today," I say out loud, surprising myself with the croakiness of my voice. I must discuss treatment for my daughter, who can't get enough oxygen, then teach inspiring piano lessons. I may be setting the bar low for my behaviour, but I really just want to get through the day without having a breakdown, especially not a sobbing, shaking fit while teaching an eleven-year-old a Diabelli sonatina.

I take one last swig of coffee and walk out the door.

* * *

"I'M SO SORRY, BUT MADELINE'S LUNGS ARE COLLAPSING. WE DID an x-ray this morning." Paul, the respiratory therapist, stares at us as he delivers his news, and we stare back.

When we first walked into the ward, residents were huddled around Dr. Lowry at the x-ray reading station, straining to see some feature. A baby's torso filled the screen; the spine, ribs, and pelvic bones are obvious. Dr. Lowry pointed to a large white patch on a lung, talking animatedly in a mysterious medical language. I tried to read the baby's name on the top corner of the screen, but I couldn't manage it without being obvious. Now we know though. That x-ray was Madeline's.

"Collapsing!" I gasp. "Why?"

"The ventilator can cause a collapsing lung, or pneumothorax, as it's called," Nurse Bridget explains. "The lung tissue is fragile and is constantly damaged by the ventilator. Eventually, the air sacs rupture and the lungs collapse."

Paul turns Madeline's respiration chart toward us. "Do you see how her oxygen needs are back to where they were when she was sick with the E. coli?" He points his stubby finger from one column to another.

"We're back to where we were last week," I whisper. "Maybe worse."

"I'm so sorry." Bridget shakes her head.

Josh exhales with frustration, then points to a machine the size and shape of a breakfast-table television. It's grey with red and yellow analog numbers on the front. Tubes flow from its back, into the incubator, like tentacles from an octopus. "New ventilator?" he asks.

"This is the jet," Paul replies as he tinkers with the settings, trying to reach an optimal calibration of oxygen, volume, frequency levels. "It's our most supportive ventilator. Instead of forcing breaths into Madeline at a normal breathing rate like the other ventilators do, it puffs tiny breaths at four times the normal rate. Basically, we are keeping Madeline's lungs constantly inflated to avoid total collapse."

I brush back the blanket from the top of incubator. Madeline looks the worst she has since birth. Her skin is gouged and scabbed from the adhesive sensors and ventilator stickers. Her stomach is oddly bloated and the layers of wrinkles that hang off her arms and neck seem even more papery-thin than before. Her entire body shakes.

"Why is she shaking, Paul?" I ask.

"It's okay. The force of the ventilator shakes the body and hopefully rattles the lungs to loosen the congestion."

"Are there downsides to this ventilator?" Josh asks.

"There are less than with other machines but, yes, all ventilators damage lungs. At least with the jet ventilator, Madeline's lungs don't have to open and close. They are constantly open so the tissues aren't as irritated. Unfortunately, a lot of air is being forced into her stomach, which causes bloating. It will become difficult to tell if she has gut issues or if there's air in her stomach."

"Don't worry about the air," Bridget says, waving her hand. "I can syringe some of it out. What you have to think about, Mom and Dad, is whether or not you'll consider treatment because we can't turn up the oxygen level much higher."

"What are our options?" I ask. "Phyllis didn't say."

"There is a steroid that is extremely effective when the lungs are wet and possibly collapsing; however, there are a number of serious side effects that you need to consider before you give permission. Dr. Lowry will explain."

"Do you need to treat right away?"

"Not this morning, but soon. We still have some room on the oxygen dial but not much. Once we get to the top, there's nothing more we can do without some powerful intervention."

Ward shoes squeak on the newly washed floors. The team of doctors walks straight from the x-ray reading station to Madeline's incubator. They carry binders and iPads preloaded with x-ray images. Not one of them smiles.

"We'll start here," Dr. Lowry says.

She is a new doctor to us. Obviously pregnant, she looks grateful when one of the residents spins a wheeled chair her way. She adjusts the chair until it's at a comfortable height to the small, spindly-wheeled writing table that her binder rests on.

"I'm Dr. Sarah Lowry." She nods in our directions. "I'm the neonatologist on call for the next two weeks, if I don't go into labour first. I have familiarized myself with Madeline's complex case with the assistance of Dr. Fiala's case notes. I believe I understand the challenges we face. Bridget, Paul—shall we begin?"

Bridget recites the now-familiar litany of statistics: gestational age, corrected age, weight, temperature, skin tone, urine and stool output, and blood work results. Paul details the change of ventilators and describes Madeline's rising oxygen requirements, and a neonatology fellow summarizes the most recent heart and abdominal ultrasounds. Dr. Lowry nods throughout, occasionally jotting notes in her binder.

"Okay," she says, "from what we've just seen on Madeline's lung x-ray, there is a partial collapse on the upper right lobe. Her blood work is clear of infection, but the lung secretions are infected. That means pneumonia. Changing her to the jet ventilator was a good move, but we have to consider other options. There are some powerful steroids available to us, but—Mom and Dad—you need to know their side effects before we even consider using them. That is imperative. I have literature for you to review today and perhaps we can talk tomorrow morning at nine?"

"Of course." I accept the fistful of leaflets from her.

"Excellent. Until then, I want physiotherapy on her chest with every handling." Again, she turns to us. "We have an instrument we use to tap the chest walls. It loosens up the mucus. Bridget, do you have one to show them?"

Bridget produces an oddly shaped pink thing resembling a rubber stamp. "Just like that," she says, thumping the apparatus against my hand.

"No pain for Madeline," says Dr. Lowry, "just a little shaking. Hopefully that will help the lung regain its shape. We'll monitor her closely throughout the day and will chat tomorrow. Questions?"

We shake our heads, grateful these people have ideas how to help Madeline. It's hard for us to consider the larger picture of her health, distracted as we are by the frequent alarms and her shocking appearance.

"Until tomorrow…" Dr. Lowry pushes off against the floor with one foot, spinning her chair in the direction of the next baby.

• • •

Day 10

"WHAT I NEED FROM YOU IS CLEAR DIRECTION HOW YOU WANT US to proceed," Dr. Lowry presses.

We're back in the family counselling room, sunk into worn-out couch cushions, holding hands and bracing ourselves for things we desperately do not want to hear.

I hold Dr. Lowry's pamphlet so tightly that the pages tear around the edges. "Bronchopulmonary Dysplasia and Your Baby" is one of the most terrifying things I've ever read. Lungs that won't clear, tissues forever scarred, drugs that cause more damage—every dire thing spelled out in black and white.

"Madeline has wet, inflamed, infected and partially collapsed lungs," the doctor continues. "A number of things caused this. The first, of course, was her extremely premature birth. Her underdeveloped lungs had to start processing air before they were ready and have been constantly damaged by the ventilator since then. The E. coli infection also placed a great strain on Madeline's body and exhausted her. Now her lung secretions are testing positive for infection, which means pneumonia. The result of all these factors is that Madeline is essentially drowning in her own lungs."

The doctor pauses, tapping her fingers against her knee as if to punctuate the rhythm of her thoughts.

"It won't matter how high we turn the ventilator pressure or the oxygen saturation level, she will not get enough air now. We have limited options. We can do nothing, and by nothing I mean we continue with antibiotics in hopes that the infection clears, keep her on the jet ventilator so her lungs stay open, and give her a dose of Lasix to help drain her lungs. Or we can do all of those things but also give her a steroid treatment. The steroid clears lungs miraculously, but it also has potential side effects. In the short term, these can include a suppressed adrenal gland and a thickening of the heart muscles. Both issues can be dealt with; however, the long-term side effects are much more concerning. Studies show that this steroid treatment greatly increases the risk of cerebral palsy. We used to use this drug like candy in the NICU, but the follow-up studies discovered debilitating neurological damage in the patient population."

"Have you changed the way you use the drug?" Josh asks.

"Indeed we have. We now use less drug for shorter periods, but Madeline would still be at risk. You might not know until she's old enough to walk or talk if there's been damage, but—let me put it to you this way—right now Madeline's oxygen level is too low and her carbon dioxide level is too high. Her lungs crackle and their secretions are infected. She isn't growing and her risk of mortality is high.

We can give her a little more oxygen but beyond that, we have very few options. You need to understand there are risks of both giving her the drug and doing nothing. We're merely days, if not hours, away from being in a really bad place."

The doctor leans forward and unbuttons the cardigan that strains her belly. I wonder what pregnancy must be like for a neonatologist. As each week of her pregnancy goes by, does she thank her lucky stars she hasn't given birth to one of the woefully sick babies she's caring for?

The doctor takes a deep breath, then presses again, "I need clear direction about how you want us to proceed."

"I think we need to talk," I say, stalling.

"Of course. You don't need to make the decision this minute, but you need to soon. We don't have much time." Dr. Lowry hauls herself out of the chair—"We'll be in touch"—then leaves us.

"This is so grim," I whisper, turning to look out the window at the uninspiring view: dirty cars, slush puddles, naked trees. "I feel that no matter what decision we make, it will be the wrong one. But, after all we've been through, it would be unbelievable to lose her to a puddle of water in her lungs."

I swallow hard, trying not to cry. I'm so tired of crying. I don't want tears. I want direction, some sign to appear, some voice to tell us what to do. But nothing comes. All I hear is the hum of the ventilation system, the crackle of a distant intercom announcement.

Josh stares at the faded wallpaper border of teddy bears and lettered blocks endlessly circling the room. "You know we have do it," he finally says, flatly. "What else can we do? The risks won't matter if she dies otherwise."

"Oh, Josh!" I pull him close and feel his chest heave with the silent, chunky sobs. He's been so strong, so calm and quiet when I've melted down, but even he has his limit.

"She's so sick!" he whispers. "That oxygen dial—did you see it? It's almost at the top. She's going to die."

"No. No." I stroke his head in little circles, kissing his forehead. "She's not going to die. We're not going to let her. We're going to keep trying and, even if she's damaged, we'll keep fighting. We won't give up."

I speak more confidently than I feel. In one moment, I accept her death. In the next, it horrifies me. I can't go by my instincts. Too many things have proven them wrong.

Josh wipes his eyes, sighs, then checks the time. "We need to go. I've got to get to work. They'll call us when they need to."

We step out into the hall, past a bulletin board of correspondence from parents. Photo cards of babies' first-year parties, computer-typed essays intended to encourage other parents, handwritten thank-you notes to the staff—some items celebrate discharges; others remember tragically short lives spent in these four walls. I choose to ignore the analogies to small angels in heaven and larger, caregiving ones on earth. I don't have the emotional energy.

Josh and I go back to peek at Madeline. I notice the oxygen percentage on the ventilator is turned up higher than it was a few minutes earlier, but I don't mention it to Josh.

"Did you get all your questions answered?" Nurse Bridget asks.

"I think so," I say. "We'll do steroids. Call when you need permission."

"We will."

Madeline's oxygen saturation alarm starts to ring, so Bridget twists the oxygen level on the ventilator a bit higher, almost to the top of the dial. I refuse to walk away until Madeline's stats are reading perfectly, so we wait for the percentage on the screen to recover and then we leave.

We make our way down the hallways of the obstetrical ward, past a young couple at Triage, she clutching her stomach, both of them grimacing. We step around toddlers wearing cheerful "Big Brother" or "Big Sister" T-shirts. We avoid the grandparents carrying balloons with welcome messages. We walk out of the hospital to our car in dead silence, isolated, yet connected by the one thing that consumes us both.

Five or six months ago, Madeline didn't even exist outside of our imaginations; she wasn't even a chemical reaction or a miniscule embryo. Her soul was somewhere—God knows where—waiting to be born, but now she's here. Wee and broken, she has a life story ahead of her, and I desperately want her to be around for it. There are so many things I can picture her doing: running barefoot in the soft June grass, dogpaddling in a cold lake, road-tripping across the country, dripping globs of sticky ice cream down mosquito-bitten arms. Her future flourishes in my mind and I'll live every minute of it whether or not she survives. I'll always know how old she'd be. I'll always picture what could have been. But right now my dreams have come to a screeching halt, kept at bay by wet, infected, half-formed lungs.

In the grand scheme of things, our problems are insignificant. Lost babies and mourning mothers have filled history. The theme is as old as life itself. Even praying for Madeline's life seems selfish. She was born sixteen weeks early. What do I think is going to happen? Her lungs are going to be damaged and she's going to become incredibly ill, then she's going to die. Die. That's it. Done.

I want to pound my fist on the car dash and cry, "God! Why are you making her suffer? Why? She's so tiny! Why does she have to be the one that suffers?"

But I don't cry and pound and yell at God. I watch trees go by, their early buds starting to bloom over the top of the car. I don't think I've ever noticed how painful the coming of spring is. All that raw beauty, growing out of nothing. It hurts the soul.

• • •

I'M TEACHING LATER THAT AFTERNOON WHEN JOSH CALLS.

"Madeline's oxygen level was turned up as high as it could go," he says in a tired, defeated voice. "Her oxygen saturation was dropping down to 30, so I gave permission. They're doing the steroids."

I sigh a long sigh at the face in hall mirror. It's a sad face. The eyes stare back like they're not actually seeing anything.

"It had to be done," I say, glancing over my shoulder at a bored nine-year-old swinging her legs on the piano bench. I want to grieve but there is no time.

"I'll call our parents," Josh says. "Dr. Lowry says Madeline's in bad shape."

"Should we go in?"

"They said they'd call again if she deteriorates further."

"I have to go, Love."

I beep the phone off and return to teaching, but I can't remember what I was thinking about before the phone rang. Rhythm? Phrasing? Oh yes, incorrect fingering at measure seventeen is creating a gap in the melody line.

I try to focus, but I can only think of Madeline. The steroid treatment feels like a last-ditch attempt, as if we're saving her life by endangering it. And what if it doesn't work? Or even if it does, what if she never lives a normal life? I like to think that even if Madeline has disabilities we will give her the best possible childhood. We will do everything we can for her. We will be strong.

Eventually the last student of the day disappears, and I charge off to the hospital, picking up Josh on the way. We rush into the NICU, expecting to see panicked nurses and rock-bottom numbers but, to our amazement, Madeline's oxygen saturation is in the high eighties. The ventilator's oxygen dial is turned down. No alarms ring. The room is utterly calm.

Nurse Bridget's eyes shine and her chin shakes a little. "She's remarkably better since we gave her the steroid. I think we may have just saved her!" she whispers.

Chapter 20

"I NEED YOUR HELP, AMY." NURSE BRITTANY POINTS TO A STACK of fresh linens on the counter. "It's time to change Madeline's bedding," she says.

Madeline is still shrivelled. The E. coli infection and pneumonia kept her hovering at the edge of life and death for too long. She's hardly gained any weight, but we have begun to hope.

"What do I do?" I ask.

"When I say go, you're going to open the door on your side of the incubator and lift Madeline straight up. I'll replace the bedding and then you'll set her back down. Don't worry about the ventilator line. I'll keep it from kinking."

Tall, commanding, fresh out of university, Brittany exudes confidence. She doesn't panic easily, no matter how many times Madeline's oxygenation alarm rings or how low the numbers go. She does what's needed, poker face intact, breathtakingly fearless. She could probably manage a linen change on her own, but she knows I haven't held Madeline yet. Madeline responds so poorly to handling—oxygen saturation plummeting, heart rate skyrocketing—that I rarely touch her. Even cupping her foot in my hand is enough to make her arms flail and the alarms ring.

"Are you sure it's okay?" I ask Brittany nervously.

"Absolutely," she says. "Are you ready?"

I nod, then reach my freshly washed hands through the circular incubator doors, into the sauna-like substitute for my womb. Brittany opens the doors on her side and lifts Madeline off the mattress. She eases Madeline into my hands, her bottom in my left hand, her head and shoulders in my right. Even without stretching my hands to their fullest reach, I can easily lift Madeline and hardly notice her weight. She is now just over a pound, a sack of loose, limp body parts, splayed at odd angles.

As I suspend Madeline a few inches above the mattress, Brittany navigates the chaos of the incubator with the finesse of a choreographed dancer, tossing used blankets into a laundry bag, rolling clean hand towels into a perfectly shaped nest, untangling a snarl of feeding tube, IV, and heart rate sensor lines.

With the incubator doors open, the inside air temperature drops, prompting an alarm to ring. As the piercing fills the air, Madeline's breathing slackens and her ventilator alarm begins ringing at a slightly higher, more insistent pitch than the first alarm. Brittany silences both alarms with her elbows, keeping her hands sanitary, but the baby in the neighbouring incubator stops breathing, so his alarm system lights up like a howling, blinking Christmas tree. His nurse scrambles to wash her hands in case she needs to fling open the incubator doors and adjust a wayward oxygen line.

The noise upsets Madeline, so her oxygen saturation plummets. Ventilated or not, she's short of air. As her oxygen saturation drops sixty percentage points down to a dangerous thirty-two, her oxygen monitor flips into its high-pitched emergency alarm. Then, her heart rate skyrockets to 220 beats per minute, triggering yet another alarm. The cacophony continues as Brittany signals for me to lay Madeline into the fresh bedding. She carefully arranges the wires and tubing across the mattress—no kinks in the ventilator tube, no pulling on the PICC line—and quickly changes Madeline's Blackberry-sized diaper. I stroke Madeline's miniscule hand for a second, then close the incubator doors on my side. Brittany does the same on hers and we wait for Madeline to settle.

It takes a few minutes, but Madeline's oxygen saturation percentage returns to the eighties and her heart rate calms to 200 beats per minute. The incubator reheats itself and the baby in the neighbouring incubator breathes again. The room falls silent and Brittany and I smile at each other in relief.

My interaction with Madeline was hardly a moment of maternal bonding, but I'm grateful for it. It was our first real physical contact since her birth and, for once, I feel useful. Usually, I feel like an observer in the NICU. From the first day, I've let someone else care for my child. I've asked permission to touch, to hold. I've taken information, not given it, and all that would have been easier to accept if the same nurse was always at the bedside, but it's not. Every twelve hours, the shift changes and a new nurse is on. I began to pray for legible handwriting the day I realized Madeline's medical chart was her only consistent caregiver.

As Madeline settles back to sleep, I blow goodnight kisses and hope she understands how much I love her despite any evidence of my existence in her world. She doesn't hear my voice from inside of me anymore, and perhaps she doesn't remember its sound. She can't possibly know my smell and she has never felt my warmth. I like to think that her sixth sense, some primal, internal voice, is shouting at her to keep fighting, keep trying, keep clawing, because I can't say a word to her, not without her breathing stopping and heart rate rising. And it isn't worth the panic.

• • •

Day 33

JOSH AND I ARE ON AN EVENING VISIT WHEN NURSE DONNA RE-ports that Madeline fluttered her eyelashes earlier in the day.

Madeline's eyes have been fused since birth like a little kitten's. Seeing her eyes might be some way for us to connect with her, some means to prove we exist.

With no small excitement, we perch on two high stools at the incubator, our noses all but pressed to the Plexiglas wall. We watch for at least an hour, but there's nothing, not even a flicker of an eyelash. Perhaps Madeline is exhausted from her earlier triumph, for she sleeps the sleep of the unborn.

"Maybe tomorrow," Donna consoles.

The next morning, the rising sun shines through the east-facing NICU windows as Josh and I again toss our coats on the window shelf and pull chairs close to the incubator. We lift the blanket, then gasp in pleasure, for there they are.

Two blue eyes—the deepest shade of blue I've ever seen, like saskatoon berries hidden in the shadows on a low branch, or summer rain clouds darkened by the setting sun. Madeline gazes steadily at us as if to say, "Who are you? What's happened to me?"

It's all too much. Josh and I hold hands and choke back tears.

"This wasn't what we had planned, Sweetheart!" we whisper. "We're so sorry—for the needles, for that ventilator tube down your throat, for those awful sensors ripping skin off you. We're so sorry!"

She blinks her lashes, lovely long things that flicker over our only window into her soul. I wish she could smile, coo, and say she forgives us, but she doesn't. She just looks pitiful and frail.

Nurse Donna smiles at us. "Would you like to hold her, Amy?"

"Can I?" I gasp.

"For a little while. We'll be super careful."

I can hardly believe the offer, so I stand in the middle of the room, stunned, wondering what to do next. Donna points to a rocking chair and Josh drags it close to the incubator. I sit down and unbutton my top, as Donna stacks two heated towels on my lap.

"Ready?" she asks.

I nod, too nervous to speak.

Donna moves quickly, unlatching the entire wall of the incubator, then sweeping all the lines into one hand while lifting Madeline with the other. She drapes the lines over my shoulder and tucks Madeline between my soft, warm breasts. I hold Madeline's folded legs against her tiny bottom with my right hand and press a warm towel over her thin back with my left. Donna fastens all the lines to my shirt with a long piece of surgical tape, then refastens the incubator door.

Still the size of a newborn golden retriever pup, Madeline stirs, pulling her head back as if she wants to look around. Her eyes roll haphazardly around their sockets as her head flops back down against my chest. Her head rests just below my collarbone so, if I tuck my chin tightly, I can see her tiny face. It is unbelievable that a face as small and scruffy as hers belongs to a living, breathing human. She looks like a tornado-swept doll found along the side of the road when the wind and rain have finally stopped. She's dearly loved, but deeply damaged.

Her oxygen saturation alarms starts to ring, so I watch the numbers on the overhead monitor, hoping we're not upsetting her.

"Watch her, Amy, not the monitor," Donna soothes. I'm keeping track."

I try to relax. I don't want Madeline to feel the tension seething through my every pore, but it is difficult to keep my heart from racing and my shoulders from rising.

"Isn't this a special moment?" Donna asks.

I smile and say, "Oh yes," but I don't feel that way. Frankly, I feel the loss and the fear all over again. Why did this have to happen? Why do I feel so horrible as I hold my daughter for the first time? I want to put her back into the incubator until she's stronger, less terrifying.

"It will get better, Amy." Donna crouches down to my level as tears fill my eyes. "I know in many ways this is tremendously sad. Holding your baby for the first time is supposed to be a happy thing, and this is stressful. But you don't have to love this because you will later. Madeline is getting stronger, bit by bit, every day. Yes, she's got many things ahead of her. We've got to get her breathing on her own, and that will take months. We've got to get her weaned off the feeding line. She'll likely require an eye surgery; maybe even a heart surgery. But one day you will walk out of here with a healthy child. I promise you."

I nod, unbelieving.

Chapter 21

TODAY IS THE DAY. IT'S HAPPENING. MADELINE IS ACTUALLY coming home.

It's July 10th, one day after her original due date. She has survived E. coli, pneumonia, an inflamed bowel, a heart murmur, innumerable apnea spells and subsequent resuscitations, wildly fluctuating heart rates, difficult eye examinations, an eventual eye surgery, constant blood work and an MRI to investigate excessive fluid in her brain. Improvements happened gradually, sometimes followed by setbacks, but over four months in hospital Madeline's body finished growing to the size it should have been at birth.

Now, at six pounds, she drinks from a bottle, has chubby cheeks, and actually looks like a baby. We know she's not in perfect condition, but we have a list of follow-up appointments as long as our arm and a pediatrician on call. It'll be okay.

Over the course of Madeline's 112 days in hospital, Josh and I made 224 visits. We drove 10,000 kilometres and completely wore out our aging car. Now, on discharge day, we drive a new, navy blue Ford with a baby seat in the back.

It's been a long journey, and at some points it felt endless. But we've grown used to the hospital and its quirks. We now know which doors are locked on weekends and when the line is shortest at the Second Cup. We covet certain parking spots—getting one close to the exit in the covered part, nearest the stairwell, has become a minor obsession for us. We analyze the fluctuating traffic levels on the Queensway, one drive after another—"A bit heavy for a Friday afternoon on a long weekend, wouldn't you say?"—and feel the ebb and flow of city life, day after day—"A hockey game at Scotiabank

Place; that explains it." We observe nuances in Madeline's care. During the weekdays, for example, on-call neonatologists have aggressive treatment strategies but, during the weekends, on-call pediatric fellows seem to have the goal of keeping the babies alive until Monday morning when the neonatologists return.

We learn the names of seventy-five nurses, and they become our biggest cheerleaders, celebrating all of Madeline's milestones—a body weight of one kilogram, her first suck on a bottle, her first day without oxygen. Some nurses are assigned to Madeline so frequently we know more about their lives than about our friends' lives—"How did your daughter's dance recital go? Did you finish the costume in time? Oh, and did you find those potted canna lilies at Home Depot I was telling you about? Good price, eh?" We keep track of their news—Tall Sheila got engaged, Short Sheila bought a townhouse, Connie vacationed in Nashville, Ruth laid turf—possibly because our own lives are stuck in one place, one room, one incubator. Chatting with them is a vicarious excursion into normalcy.

But as impossible as it may have seemed earlier, discharge day is here.

The nurses have taught us how to feed Madeline slowly from a tiny bottle so she has time to breathe. We've practised bathing her in a bathtub no bigger than my six-quart slow cooker, holding her in our arms, covering her with a towel as we wash her with a warm cloth. She still seems fragile, but her neck muscles are stronger than a newborn's. She can very nearly hold up her head, which seems freakishly talented for a mini-baby like her.

One day, months ago, when Madeline was sick with pneumonia, I bought a newborn-size white lace dress. I bought it with faith and called it her discharge dress. Now, I pull off Madeline's preemie-size sleeper and slip the dress over her head. I balance her chin between my thumb and second finger. Her eyes bulge open at this change of position and her tongue laps her lips. I dress her carefully, feeding her arms through the sleeves as if I might break her, then lift her off her crib and ease her into the car seat. All of the car seat lines are pulled to their shortest setting, so we stuff blankets around her tiny head to keep it from lolling. With gentle hands, Josh fastens the straps around her, chatting amicably as if she's an adult—"Oh, we're so pleased you're coming home, Baby. So pleased."

We load all our things into a plus-size wheelchair—breast pumping supplies, a musical crib mobile, and a suitcase full of Madeline's doll-sized clothes. We strip the work station around Madeline's crib of its memorabilia—a certificate to celebrate the day Madeline reached one kilogram, Josh's and my work schedules, a party hat made by the nurses for Madeline to wear on Josh's recent thirtieth birthday. We're removing our claim on this space, our ownership of this little corner of the hospital. Our right to come and go freely is over.

It's time for us to leave, but everything feels ceremonial, as if a soundtrack is playing somewhere; the credits are about to roll.

We walk through the NICU, past the resuscitation table, past the first incubator where Madeline lay struggling and fighting and hardly living at all. It's a victory lap—our child has beaten the odds—but we eye the family meeting room with sadness and nervously slip past the x-ray viewing station. We say one more round of goodbyes, but the nurses have already turned to their next tasks. Madeline's sheets have been stripped off her crib; her paperwork is already on a cart destined for the archives. The NICU has moved on and so must we.

Josh carries Madeline's seat and I push the wheelchair filled with our things down the hallway. We take the elevator for the last time, then stroll out of the hospital into the bright summer sunshine. People smile and nod in our direction, probably assuming our baby was just born, and we beam at each other as if we're pulling off a daring heist. We're taking her home! Madeline! The baby who was too small to touch. The micro-preemie who for weeks and weeks couldn't be unplugged from machines, not even for a minute. That baby! We're taking her home.

Despite nature conspiring against us, so many things worked for us—ventilators, antibiotics, steroids, a medical team that never lost hope, the public health policies that valued Madeline's life over the enormous costs required to sustain it. But more than that, there were intangible things which couldn't be funded or researched into existence. Madeline's will to live, her tenacity to survive—these are the answers to our prayers, the miracles we rejoice in.

We reach the car, and I click Madeline's seat into its base, then ease the door shut behind me. Madeline sleeps, her eyes scrunched shut against the daylight. She's so perfect. All the scars have healed on her face, just a few remain out of sight under her dress. If you didn't know her story, there would be no reason to suspect her history.

My cellphone vibrates in my bag and I pull it out to see Mom's number on the call display. I hit the answer button and whisper, "Hey."

"Is it happening?" she whispers back.

"It's happening," I say. And that's all I say, because we're both crying. We're crying for the morning I nearly gave birth at home, for the counselling sessions, for the ultrasounds, for the continual resuscitations, for the infections, for the surgery, for all the moments when death seemed inevitable.

Josh turns around from the front seat. "Are you ready, Love?"

"Yep," I say. "Let's get out of here."

•   •   •

A Year Later

"AMY, COME QUICKLY!" JOSH CALLS.

I run into the living room to see Madeline perching on her tiptoes, giggling and drooling around her first two teeth. I lunge for the camera from the side table and drop to the floor.

"Ready!" I say, pressing the record button. The red light flashes and, as if on cue, Madeline steps toward us. Arms stretched wide for balance, she teeters and totters haphazardly, but she does it. On the anniversary of her hospital discharge, she walks.

Josh and I cheer, "Yay, Baby! You can do it! Well done!" But we're crying too, crying from relief. Seeing Madeline walk affirms our greatest hopes for her. To be healthy, and strong, and enjoying life— that's all we've ever wanted. If she can walk, what can't she do?

• • •

MADELINE IS A NOW HEALTHY LITTLE GIRL. SHE HAS SPARKLY BLUE eyes, a quick and ready temper, and an infectious giggle. She learned her first word—"dog"—on the Katimavik walking path one beautiful summer afternoon. She's fearless. She's reckless. She's funny.

Acknowledgements

What began as a cathartic journaling of Madeline's birth turned into something far bigger and I thank all the friends and family members who got excited about this book early on. Thank you, Allison Smith, for questioning every metaphor and slashing unnecessary words; Jeff LaRose, for pointing out my insatiable desire to add commas; Linda Meyer, for challenging the details of my memory; Beth Groulx, for correcting my medical knowledge; and Janet Boyes and Betty Esler, for carefully catching errors. Thank you, Karen Haughian, for seeing the potential in my writing and for taking on this project. Lastly, thank you, Josh Boyes, for being a wonderful partner in life and father to Madeline. Without your support, this book would not have been written.

I have tried to recreate events and conversations from my memories of them. In order to maintain the anonymity of health care professionals, I have changed the names of individuals and hospitals.

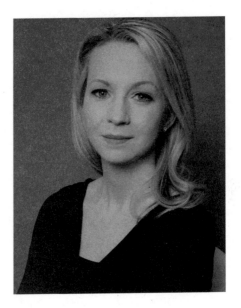

About the Author

AMY BOYES MAKES HER HOME IN OTTAWA, ONTARIO, WITH HER husband, Josh, and their daughter, Madeline. A pianist and an educator, Amy earned music degrees at Brandon University in Manitoba and the University of Alberta in Edmonton, and performance and pedagogy diplomas from the Royal Conservatory of Music in Toronto (RCM) and Trinity College in London, UK. As a music festival adjudicator and examiner for RCM, Amy enjoys connecting with young performers throughout Canada. She is also an active volunteer with the Ontario Registered Music Teachers' Association. When not teaching in her busy piano studio, or chasing after Madeline, Amy carves out a few minutes, every day, for writing. Her work can be found in a variety of sources such as *The American Music Teacher's Magazine* or *The Humber Literary Review*.

www.micromiracle-story.com